Procedure Checklists to Accompany
Rosdahl & Kowalski's

Textbook of
Basic Nursing

EIGHTH EDITION

Marjorie L. Roark, RN, BSN, MEd
Nurse Educator
Department of Professional Development
University of Chicago Hospitals
Chicago, Illinois

Visit the Lippincott Williams & Wilkins Website
http://www.lww.com

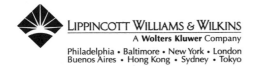
LIPPINCOTT WILLIAMS & WILKINS
A **Wolters Kluwer** Company
Philadelphia • Baltimore • New York • London
Buenos Aires • Hong Kong • Sydney • Tokyo

Ancillary Editor: Doris Wray
Senior Production Editor: Rosanne Hallowell
Senior Production Manager: Helen Ewan
Managing Editor / Production: Erika Kors
Art Director: Carolyn O'Brien
Manufacturing Manager: William Alberti
Compositor: Lippincott Williams & Wilkins
Printer: Victor Graphics

Eighth Edition

9 8 7 6 5 4 3 2 1

ISBN 0-7817-3715X

Care has been taken to confirm the accuracy of the information presented and to describe generally accepted practices. However, the author, editors, and publisher are not responsible for errors or omissions or for any consequences from application of the information in this book and make no warranty, express or implied, with respect to the content of the publication.

The author, editors, and publisher have exerted every effort to ensure that drug selection and dosage set forth in this text are in accordance with the current recommendations and practice at the time of publication. However, in view of ongoing research, changes in government regulations, and the constant flow of information relating to drug therapy and drug reactions, the reader is urged to check the package insert for each drug for any change in indications and dosage and for added warnings and precautions This is particularly important when the recommended agent is a new or infrequently employed drug.

Some drugs and medical devices presented in this publication have Food and Drug Administration (FDA) clearance for limited use in restricted research settings. It is the responsibility of the health care provider to ascertain the FDA status of each drug or device planned for use in his or her clinical practice.

LWW.com

Introduction

Developing clinical competency is a major challenge for each fundamentals student. To facilitate the mastery of nursing procedures, we are happy to provide *Procedure Checklists to Accompany Rosdahl & Kowalski's Textbook of Basic Nursing, 8th edition*. The Procedure Checklists follow each step of the procedure to provide a complete evaluative tool. Students can use the checklists to facilitate self evaluation, and faculty will find them useful in measuring and recording student performance. Three-hole punched and perforated, these checklists can be easily reproduced and brought to the simulation laboratory or clinical area.

The checklists are designed to record an evaluation of each step of the procedure:
- A check mark in the "E" (excels) column indicates that this is a skill they are excellent at performing.
- A check mark in the "S" (satisfactory) column indicates use of the recommended technique.
- A check mark in the "N.P." (needs practice) column indicate use of *some but not all* of each recommended technique.

The comments section allows you to highlight suggestions that will improve skills. Space is available at the bottom of each checklist to record final pass/fail evaluation, date, and the signature of the student and evaluating faculty member.

Contents

NURSING PROCEDURES

Additional Procedure Checklists can be found on http://connection.lww.com

Inserting a Nasogastric Tube

SUPPLIES AND EQUIPMENT

✔ Gloves
✔ Nasogastric tube
✔ Water-soluble substance (K-Y jelly)
✔ Protective towel covering for client
✔ Emesis basin
✔ Tape for marking placement and securing tube

✔ Glass of water (if allowed)
✔ Straw for glass of water
✔ Stethoscope
✔ 60 mL catheter-tip syringe
✔ Rubber band and safety pin
✔ Suction equipment or tube feeding equipment

RECOMMENDED TECHNIQUE	E	S	NP	Comments
1. Gather equipment and supplies.	☐	☐	☐	_____
2. Check the physician's order, and determine the type, size, and purpose of the NG tube.	☐	☐	☐	_____
3. Check client's identity band.	☐	☐	☐	_____
4. Obtain NG suction equipment or NG tube feeding equipment as required.	☐	☐	☐	_____
5. Set up tube feeding equipment or suction equipment, and test to make sure it functions properly.	☐	☐	☐	_____
6. Instruct the client in the procedure and assess his or her capabilities of cooperating with the procedure.	☐	☐	☐	_____
5. Wash hands. Put on gloves.	☐	☐	☐	_____
6. Position client in full Fowler's position if possible.	☐	☐	☐	_____
7. Place a clean towel over the client's chest as a bib-type protection.	☐	☐	☐	_____
8. Measure the length of the tube that will be needed to reach the stomach.	☐	☐	☐	_____
9. With a damp washcloth, wipe the client's face and nose. Do not use soap. It may be necessary to wipe the outside of the nose with an alcohol wipe. Be sure to cover the eyes with a small, dry towel or washcloth when wiping down the exterior of the nose with an alcohol wipe.	☐	☐	☐	_____
10. Protect the eyes from any alcohol fumes from the alcohol wipe by briefly covering them with a cloth.	☐	☐	☐	_____
11. Ask the client if he or she has difficulty breathing out of one of the nares. Test for naris obstructions by closing one nostril and then the other and asking the client to breath through the nose for each attempt. If the client has difficulty breathing out of one naris but not the other, try to insert the NG tube in that naris.	☐	☐	☐	_____

RECOMMENDED TECHNIQUE (*Continued*)	E	S	NP	Comments

12. Put on gloves and apply water-soluble lubricant to 4 to 8 inches of the tube. ☐ ☐ ☐ _____

13. With the client sitting up, flex the head forward. Tilt the tip of the nose upward, and insert the tube gently into the nose to as far as the back of the throat. Guide the tube straight back. ☐ ☐ ☐ _____

14. When the tube reaches the nasopharynx, stop briefly and have the client lower his or her head slightly. ☐ ☐ ☐ _____

15. Ask the client to swallow as the tube is advanced. Advance the tube several times as the client swallows until the correct marked position on the tube is reached. ☐ ☐ ☐ _____

16. If coughing, persistent gagging, cyanosis, or dyspnea occurs, remove the tube immediately. ☐ ☐ ☐ _____

17. If obstruction is felt, pull out the tube and try the other naris. ☐ ☐ ☐ _____

18. Encourage the client to breathe through his or her mouth. ☐ ☐ ☐ _____

19. Have the client or the assistant hold the glass of water with the straw. Keep an emesis basin and tissues handy. ☐ ☐ ☐ _____

20. Insert the tube as far as the pre-marked insertion point. Place a temporary piece of tape across the nose and tube. ☐ ☐ ☐ _____

21. Check the back of the client's throat to make sure that the tube is not curled in the back of the throat. ☐ ☐ ☐ _____

22. Check the tube for correct placement by at least two and preferably three of the following methods: ☐ ☐ ☐ _____

    a. Aspirate stomach contents. Stomach aspirate will appear cloudy, green, tan, off-white, bloody, or brown. It is not always possible to see the difference between stomach and respiratory aspirates. ☐ ☐ ☐ _____

    b. Check pH of aspirate. The pH of stomach aspirate is considered more accurate than visual inspection. Stomach aspirate generally has a pH range of 0 to 6, commonly less than 4. The aspirate of respiratory contents is generally more alkaline with a pH of 7 or more. ☐ ☐ ☐ _____

RECOMMENDED TECHNIQUE (*Continued*)	E	S	NP	Comments
c. Inject 30 mL of air into the stomach, and listen with the stethoscope for the "whoosh" of air into the stomach. The small diameters of some NG tubes may make it difficult to hear air entering the stomach.	☐	☐	☐	_____
d. Confirm by x-ray placement. X-ray visualization is the only method that is considered positive.	☐	☐	☐	_____
23. Once stomach placement has been confirmed, tape the tube using prepared tape strips or a commercial NG securing tape.	☐	☐	☐	_____
24. Clean the client's area and position the client for comfort.	☐	☐	☐	_____
25. To prevent aspiration of stomach contents during NG tube feedings, the head of the bed must remain elevated at 30 degrees or more at all times.	☐	☐	☐	_____
26. Chart the procedure stating the date, time, type, and size of NG tube used; left or right naris; amount and type of aspirate; suction or feeding started; and client response to the procedure. It is not uncommon to have slight bleeding from irritation of the mucosa in the nose. Any trauma or difficulty during the procedure needs to be charted, documented, and observed.	☐	☐	☐	_____
27. After the procedure, chart and monitor the type and amount of suction used. Each shift, monitor and record the suction in mmHg and the amount and type of aspirate.	☐	☐	☐	_____
28. Monitor intake and output.	☐	☐	☐	_____
29. Always confirm placement of the NG tube prior to insertion of medications, application of suction, or instillation of tube feedings.	☐	☐	☐	_____

KEY: E = Excels   S = Satisfactory   NP = Needs Practice

☐ **Pass**   ☐ **Fail**

Student's Signature: _____ Date: _____

Instructor's Signature: _____ Date: _____

Administering a Tube Feeding

SUPPLIES AND EQUIPMENT

- ✔ Gloves
- ✔ Feeding pump (optional)
- ✔ Clamp (optional)
- ✔ Feeding solution
- ✔ Large catheter tip syringe (30 mL or larger)
- ✔ Other optional equipment (disposable pad, pH indicator strips, water-soluble lubricant, paper towels)
- ✔ Feeding bag with tubing
- ✔ Water
- ✔ Measuring cup

RECOMMENDED TECHNIQUE	E	S	NP	Comments
1. Gather equipment and supplies after checking the physician's order for tube feeding.	☐	☐	☐	_____
2. Prepare formula:	☐	☐	☐	_____
a. Shake can thoroughly. Check expiration date.	☐	☐	☐	_____
b. If formula is in powdered form, mix according to the instructions on the package. Prepare enough for 24 hours only. Use a large enough container for the mixed amount, and refrigerate any unused formula. Label and date the container. Allow formula to reach room temperature before using.	☐	☐	☐	_____
3. Explain the procedure to the client.	☐	☐	☐	_____
4. Wash hands prior to putting on gloves.	☐	☐	☐	_____
5. Position the client with the head of the bed elevated at least 30 to 40 degrees.	☐	☐	☐	_____
6. Determine placement of feeding tube: a. Aspirate stomach secretions.	☐	☐	☐	_____
(1) Attach syringe to end of feeding tube.	☐	☐	☐	_____
(2) Gently pull back on plunger.	☐	☐	☐	_____
(3) Measure amount of residual fluid (clamp tube if it is necessary to remove the syringe).	☐	☐	☐	_____
(4) Return residual to stomach through tube, and continue with feeding if amount does not exceed agency protocol or physician's orders (if greater than 120 mL or no return is obtained, refer to "problem chart" in Table 32-2).	☐	☐	☐	_____

RECOMMENDED TECHNIQUE (*Continued*)	E	S	NP	Comments

b. Inject 10 to 20 mL of air into tube (3–5 mL for children). ☐ ☐ ☐ _____

  (1) Attach syringe filled with air to tube. ☐ ☐ ☐ _____

  (2) Inject air while listening with stethoscope over left upper quadrant. ☐ ☐ ☐ _____

c. Measure the pH of aspirated gastric secretions. ☐ ☐ ☐ _____

d. Take an x-ray or ultrasound (may be needed to determine tube placement). ☐ ☐ ☐ _____

Intermittent or Bolus Feeding

7. If using a feeding bag:

a. Hang the feeding bag setup 12 to 18 inches above the stomach. Clamp the tubing. Fill the bag with prescribed formula and prime the tubing by opening the clamp, allowing the feeding to flow through the tubing. Reclamp the tube. ☐ ☐ ☐ _____

b. Attach end of the setup to the gastric tube and open the damp. Adjust flow according to the physician's order. ☐ ☐ ☐ _____

c. Add 30 to 60 mL of water to the feeding bag as feeding is completed; run into a basin. Clamp the tube and disconnect the feeding setup. ☐ ☐ ☐ _____

8. If using a syringe:

a. Clamp the gastric tube. With the plunger or bulb removed, insert the tip of the large syringe into the gastric tube. Pour feeding into the syringe. Raise the syringe 12 to 18 inches above the stomach. Open the clamp. ☐ ☐ ☐ _____

b. Allow feeding to flow slowly into the stomach. Raise and lower the syringe to control the rate of flow. Add additional formula to the syringe as it empties until feeding is complete.

Continuous Feeding

9. If using a feeding pump:

a. Clamp the feeding setup and hang on pole. Add feeding solution to the bag. Open the clamp and prime the tubing. ☐ ☐ ☐ _____

RECOMMENDED TECHNIQUE (*Continued*)	E	S	NP	Comments

b. Thread the tubing through or load tubing into the pump, according to the manufacturer's specifications. Attach the end of the setup to the gastric tube. Set the prescribed rate and volume according to the manufacturer's directions. Open the clamp and turn on the pump. ☐ ☐ ☐ _____

c. Stop feeding every 4 to 8 hours and assess residual. Flush the tube every 6 to 8 hours. ☐ ☐ ☐ _____

10. Terminate feeding when completed. Instill prescribed amount of water. Keep the client's head elevated for 20 to 30 minutes. ☐ ☐ ☐ _____

11. Assess the skin around the injection site of surgically placed tubes. Cleanse skin with mild soap and water and dry thoroughly. Check site for redness, swelling, pain, or additional signs of inflammation. ☐ ☐ ☐ _____

12. Provide mouth care by brushing teeth, offering mouthwash, and keeping the lips moist. ☐ ☐ ☐ _____

13. Clean and replace equipment according to agency policy. ☐ ☐ ☐ _____

14. Remove gloves and wash hands. ☐ ☐ ☐ _____

15. Document time, amount of residual, amount of feeding, and client's reactions to feeding. ☐ ☐ ☐ _____

KEY: E = Excels   S = Satisfactory   NP = Needs Practice

☐ **Pass**   ☐ **Fail**

Student's Signature: _____ Date: _____

Instructor's Signature: _____ Date: _____

Handwashing

SUPPLIES AND EQUIPMENT
✔ Liquid or bar soap
✔ Paper towels

RECOMMENDED TECHNIQUE	E	S	NP	Comments
1. Remove jewelry. Plain wedding band may remain in place.	☐	☐	☐	_____
2. Stand in front of the sink, and avoid leaning against it.	☐	☐	☐	_____
3. Turn on the water, and regulate its flow and temperature. Knee or foot pedals may be available on some sinks. In some facilities, water automatically flows when placing hands under the faucet.	☐	☐	☐	_____
4. Wet hands and forearms with water, keeping the hands lower than elbows.	☐	☐	☐	_____
5. Apply an antibacterial liquid soap. If necessary to press a level to dispense soap, do so with a paper towel. Liquid soap with a foot-operated dispenser is the most sanitary.	☐	☐	☐	_____
6. Wash hands, wrists, and lower forearms for a minimum of 10 to 15 seconds, using a scrubbing motion. Interlace fingers and rub hands back and forth.	☐	☐	☐	_____
7. Insert fingernails from one hand under those of other hand using a sweeping motion. Repeat with the other hand.	☐	☐	☐	_____
8. Rinse thoroughly, keeping hands lower than forearms.	☐	☐	☐	_____
9. Repeat the procedure if hands are very soiled.	☐	☐	☐	_____
10. Dry hands thoroughly with a paper towel. Discard the towel.	☐	☐	☐	_____
11. Use a clean paper towel to turn off faucets.	☐	☐	☐	_____

KEY: E = Excels   S = Satisfactory   NP = Needs Practice

☐ **Pass**   ☐ **Fail**

Student's Signature: _____ Date: _____

Instructor's Signature: _____ Date: _____

Undressing the Immobile Client

SUPPLIES AND EQUIPMENT
✔ Healthcare facility gown

RECOMMENDED TECHNIQUE	E	S	NP	Comments
1. Push the client's blouse or shirt off one shoulder.	☐	☐	☐	_____
2. Roll the sleeve on the same side down to the wrist.	☐	☐	☐	_____
3. Slip off the sleeve.	☐	☐	☐	_____
4. Repeat steps 1 to 3 on the other side.	☐	☐	☐	_____
5. Put a gown on the client.	☐	☐	☐	_____
6. Unfasten the waistband, and push all lower garments as far as possible around the client's hips.	☐	☐	☐	_____
7. Ask the client to raise the hips to assist in pulling down the clothes.	☐	☐	☐	_____
8. If the client cannot raise his or her hips, request assistance from other healthcare personnel.	☐	☐	☐	_____
9. If garments must come off over the head, slip the client's arms from the sleeves, push the clothing up to the hips, and ask the client to raise the hips. Pull the garments up to the shoulders. To get clothing over the shoulders more easily, turn the client's shoulders first to one side and then to the other.	☐	☐	☐	_____
10. Slip garments over the face by raising the client's head and gathering the clothes together into a roll behind the head. Do not cover the client's face, and avoid dragging clothing over the face.	☐	☐	☐	_____
11. When putting the gown on the client, cover him or her with a bath blanket and work under it as much as possible.	☐	☐	☐	_____

KEY: E = Excels   S = Satisfactory   NP = Needs Practice

☐ **Pass**   ☐ **Fail**

Student's Signature: _____ Date: _____

Instructor's Signature: _____ Date: _____

Measuring Body Temperature

Oral Temperature by Electronic Thermometer

SUPPLIES AND EQUIPMENT
✔ Thermometer with probe
✔ Disposable probe covers
✔ Paper or flow sheet
✔ Pen

RECOMMENDED TECHNIQUE	E	S	NP	Comments
1. Gather equipment.	☐	☐	☐	_____
2. Wash hands.	☐	☐	☐	_____
3. Explain the procedure to the client.	☐	☐	☐	_____
4. Check that the oral probe is attached to the portable thermometer unit. Slide a disposable plastic cover onto the probe until it snaps into place.	☐	☐	☐	_____
5. Place the probe under the client's tongue at the base of the sublingual pocket on either side.	☐	☐	☐	_____
6. Instruct the client to close the lips (not the teeth) around the probe.	☐	☐	☐	_____
7. Remove the thermometer when a "beep" sounds or the numbers stop flashing and the digital reading of the temperature is displayed.	☐	☐	☐	_____
8. Remove the probe from the client's mouth and read the displayed temperature.	☐	☐	☐	_____
9. Push the eject button to discard the plastic probe cover into the wastebasket. Return the oral probe to the portable unit.	☐	☐	☐	_____
10. Wash hands.	☐	☐	☐	_____
11. Record the client's temperature on paper or flow sheet. Report an abnormal reading to the appropriate person.	☐	☐	☐	_____

KEY: E = Excels   S = Satisfactory   NP = Needs Practice

☐ **Pass**   ☐ **Fail**

Student's Signature: _____   Date: _____

Instructor's Signature: _____   Date: _____

NURSING PROCEDURE 46-1 *(Continued)*
Measuring Body Temperature

Oral Temperature by Glass Thermometer

SUPPLIES AND EQUIPMENT
- ✔ Thermometer with plastic wrapper
- ✔ Soft tissues
- ✔ Paper or flow sheet
- ✔ Pen

RECOMMENDED TECHNIQUE	E	S	NP	Comments
1. Gather equipment.	☐	☐	☐	_____
2. Wash hands.	☐	☐	☐	_____
3. Explain the procedure to the client.	☐	☐	☐	_____
4. Wipe the thermometer from the bulb toward fingers with a tissue.	☐	☐	☐	_____
5. Hold the thermometer firmly with thumb and forefinger; shake it with strong wrist movements until the mercury line falls to at least 35°C (95°F).	☐	☐	☐	_____
6. Place the bulb of the thermometer well under the client's tongue. Instruct the client to close the lips (not the teeth) around the bulb.	☐	☐	☐	_____
7. Remove the thermometer after 3 to 5 minutes, according to agency guidelines.	☐	☐	☐	_____
8. Remove the thermometer; wipe it once using a firm twisting motion.	☐	☐	☐	_____
9. Hold the thermometer at eye level. Read to the nearest tenth.	☐	☐	☐	_____
10. Dispose the tissue. Wash the thermometer in lukewarm, soapy water. Dry and replace the thermometer in a container at the bedside. Wash hands.	☐	☐	☐	_____
11. Record temperature on paper or flow sheet. Report an abnormal reading to the appropriate person.	☐	☐	☐	_____

KEY: E = Excels   S = Satisfactory   NP = Needs Practice

☐ **Pass**   ☐ **Fail**

Student's Signature: _____   Date: _____

Instructor's Signature: _____   Date: _____

NURSING PROCEDURE 46-1 *(Continued)*
Measuring Body Temperature

Rectal Temperature by Glass or Electronic Thermometer

SUPPLIES AND EQUIPMENT
✔ Rectal thermometer
✔ Wipes
✔ Tissues

✔ Water-soluble lubricant or lubricated probe cover
✔ Disposable gloves
✔ Graphic record and pen

RECOMMENDED TECHNIQUE	E	S	NP	Comments
1. Wash hands and put on gloves.	☐	☐	☐	_____
2. Turn the client on one side.	☐	☐	☐	_____
3. For the glass thermometer, lubricate the client's rectal area and the bulb up to 1 inch above it with lubricant on a wipe. Use a lubricated probe cover with an electronic thermometer.	☐	☐	☐	_____
4. Fold back the bedclothes, and separate the client's buttocks so that the anal opening is clearly visible.	☐	☐	☐	_____
5. As the client takes a slow, deep breath, insert the thermometer about 1.5 inches.	☐	☐	☐	_____
6. Hold the thermometer in place for 3 to 5 minutes, according to agency protocol.	☐	☐	☐	_____
7. Remove and wipe the glass thermometer toward the bulb, or dispose of the probe cover. Read the temperature.	☐	☐	☐	_____
8. Dispose of the equipment properly. Wash hands.	☐	☐	☐	_____
9. Document the temperature on the client's graphic record. Indicate that temperature was taken rectally by writing "(R)" next to it.	☐	☐	☐	_____

KEY: E = Excels   S = Satisfactory   NP = Needs Practice

☐ **Pass**   ☐ **Fail**

Student's Signature: _____ Date: _____

Instructor's Signature: _____ Date: _____

NURSING PROCEDURE 46-1 *(Continued)*
Measuring Body Temperature

Axillary Temperature by Glass or Electronic Thermometer

SUPPLIES AND EQUIPMENT
- ✔ Appropriate thermometer
- ✔ Graphic chart
- ✔ Pen

RECOMMENDED TECHNIQUE	E	S	NP	Comments
1. Wash hands.	☐	☐	☐	_____
2. Be sure the client's axilla is dry. If it is moist, pat it dry gently before inserting the thermometer.	☐	☐	☐	_____
3. After placing the probe or bulb of the thermometer into the axilla, bring the client's arm down against the body as tightly as possible, with the forearm resting across the chest.	☐	☐	☐	_____
4. Hold the glass thermometer in place for 8 to 10 minutes. Hold the electronic thermometer in place until the reading registers directly.	☐	☐	☐	_____
5. Remove and read the thermometer. Dispose of the equipment properly. Wash hands.	☐	☐	☐	_____
6. Record the reading per agency procedures. Indicate that the axillary method was used "(Ax)."	☐	☐	☐	_____

KEY: E = Excels   S = Satisfactory   NP = Needs Practice

☐ **Pass**   ☐ **Fail**

Student's Signature: _____ Date: _____

Instructor's Signature: _____ Date: _____

NURSING PROCEDURE 46-1 *(Continued)*

Measuring Body Temperature

Tympanic Temperature

SUPPLIES AND EQUIPMENT
✔ Tympanic thermometer
✔ Disposable probe cover

RECOMMENDED TECHNIQUE	E	S	NP	Comments
1. Wash hands.	☐	☐	☐	_____
2. Explain the procedure to the client.	☐	☐	☐	_____
3. Hold the probe in dominant hand. Use the client's same ear as dominant hand (eg, use the client's right ear when using right hand).	☐	☐	☐	_____
4. Select the desired mode of temperature. Use the rectal equivalent for children under 3 years of age. Wait for a "ready" message to display.	☐	☐	☐	_____
5. With nondominant hand, grasp the adult's external ear at the midpoint. Pull the external ear up and back. For a child of 6 years or younger, use nondominant hand to pull the ear down and back.	☐	☐	☐	_____
6. Slowly advance the probe into the client's ear with a back and forth motion until it seals the ear canal.	☐	☐	☐	_____
7. Point the probe's tip in an imaginary line from the client's sideburns to his or her opposite eyebrow.	☐	☐	☐	_____
8. As soon as the instrument is in correct position, press the button to activate the thermometer.	☐	☐	☐	_____
9. Keep the probe in place until the thermometer makes a sound or flashes a light.	☐	☐	☐	_____
10. Read the temperature and discard the probe cover. Replace the thermometer and wash hands.	☐	☐	☐	_____
11. Record the temperature on the client's record.	☐	☐	☐	_____

KEY: E = Excels   S = Satisfactory   NP = Needs Practice

☐ **Pass**   ☐ **Fail**

Student's Signature: _____   Date: _____

Instructor's Signature: _____   Date: _____

Measuring a Radial Pulse

SUPPLIES AND EQUIPMENT
- ✔ Watch with a second hand
- ✔ Paper or flow sheet
- ✔ Pen

RECOMMENDED TECHNIQUE	E	S	NP	Comments
1. Wash hands.	☐	☐	☐	_____
2. Explain the procedure to the client.	☐	☐	☐	_____
3. Position the client's forearm comfortably with the wrist extended and the palm down.	☐	☐	☐	_____
4. Place the tips of first, second, and third fingers over the client's radial artery on the inside of the wrist on the thumb side.	☐	☐	☐	_____
5. Press gently against the client's radial artery to the point where pulsations are distinctly felt.	☐	☐	☐	_____
6. Using a watch, count the pulse beats for 30 seconds and multiply by two to get the rate per minute.	☐	☐	☐	_____
7. Count the pulse for a full minute if it is abnormal in any way, or take an apical pulse.	☐	☐	☐	_____
8. Record the rate (BPM) on paper or the flow sheet. Report any irregular findings to the appropriate person.	☐	☐	☐	_____
9. Wash hands.	☐	☐	☐	_____

KEY: E = Excels   S = Satisfactory   NP = Needs Practice

☐ **Pass**   ☐ **Fail**

Student's Signature: _____ Date: _____

Instructor's Signature: _____ Date: _____

Counting Respirations

SUPPLIES AND EQUIPMENT
✔ Watch with second hand
✔ Paper or flow sheet
✔ Pen

RECOMMENDED TECHNIQUE	E	S	NP	Comments
1. Prepare to count respirations by keeping own fingertips on the client's pulse.	☐	☐	☐	_____
2. Observe the rise and fall of the client's chest (one inspiration and one expiration). Count respirations by placing hand lightly on the client's chest or abdomen.	☐	☐	☐	_____
a. Count respirations for 30 seconds and multiply by 2 to get the rate per minute.	☐	☐	☐	_____
b. Count respirations for 1 full minute for an infant, a young child, or an adult with an irregular, more rapid rate.	☐	☐	☐	_____
3. Record the rate on paper or the flow sheet. Report any irregular findings to the appropriate person.	☐	☐	☐	_____
4. Wash hands.	☐	☐	☐	_____

KEY: E = Excels   S = Satisfactory   NP = Needs Practice

☐ **Pass**   ☐ **Fail**

Student's Signature: _____ Date: _____

Instructor's Signature: _____ Date: _____

Measuring Blood Pressure and Measuring Orthostatic Blood Pressure

SUPPLIES AND EQUIPMENT
- ✔ Stethoscope
- ✔ Sphygmomanometer
- ✔ Blood pressure cuff (appropriate size)
- ✔ Alcohol wipe
- ✔ Paper or flow sheet
- ✔ Pen

RECOMMENDED TECHNIQUE	E	S	NP	Comments
1. Gather equipment. Select a cuff that is the appropriate size for the client. Cleanse the stethoscope's ear pieces and diaphragm with an alcohol wipe.	☐	☐	☐	_____
2. Wash hands.	☐	☐	☐	_____
3. Explain the procedure to the client.	☐	☐	☐	_____
4. Assist the client to a comfortable position. Support the selected arm; turn the palm upward. Remove any constrictive clothing.	☐	☐	☐	_____
5. Palpate the brachial artery. Center the cuff's bladder approximately 1 inch (2.5 cm) above the site where the brachial pulse is palpated.	☐	☐	☐	_____
6. Wrap the cuff snugly around the client's arm, and secure the end appropriately.	☐	☐	☐	_____
7. Check that the mercury manometer is vertical, at eye level, and level with the client's heart.	☐	☐	☐	_____
8. Palpate the radial or brachial pulse with one hand. Close the screw clamp on the bulb, and inflate the cuff while still checking the pulse with the other hand. Observe the point where pulse is no longer palpable.	☐	☐	☐	_____
9. Open the screw clamp, deflate the cuff, and wait 30 seconds.	☐	☐	☐	_____
10. Position the stethoscope's earpieces comfortably in ears (turn tips slightly forward), and place the diaphragm or bell over the client's brachial artery.	☐	☐	☐	_____
11. Close the screw clamp on the bulb and inflate the cuff to a pressure 30 mm Hg above the point where the pulse had disappeared.	☐	☐	☐	_____
12. Open the clamp and allow the mercury column or aneroid dial to fall at 2 to 3 mm Hg per second.	☐	☐	☐	_____
13. Note the point on the column or dial at which initial distinct sound is heard.	☐	☐	☐	_____

RECOMMENDED TECHNIQUE (*Continued*)	E	S	NP	Comments
14. Continue deflating the cuff, and note the point where the sound disappears.	☐	☐	☐	_____
15. Release any remaining air in the cuff and remove it. If a recheck reading is done for any reason, allow a 1-minute interval before taking blood pressure again.	☐	☐	☐	_____
16. Assist the client to a comfortable position. Advise the client of the reading.	☐	☐	☐	_____
17. Wash hands.	☐	☐	☐	_____
18. Record results on paper or the flow sheet. Write the systolic pressure over the diastolic (using even numbers). For example, record a systolic of 120 and a diastolic of 70 as 120/70. Indicate site where the blood pressure was taken. Report any irregular findings.	☐	☐	☐	_____

KEY: E = Excels   S = Satisfactory   NP = Needs Practice

☐ **Pass**   ☐ **Fail**

Student's Signature: _____ Date: _____

Instructor's Signature: _____ Date: _____

Turning the Client to a Side-Lying Position

SUPPLIES AND EQUIPMENT
✔ Pillows
✔ Side rails
✔ Cotton blanket or towels, rolled for support

RECOMMENDED TECHNIQUE	E	S	NP	Comments
1. Wash hands.	☐	☐	☐	_____
2. Explain the procedure to the client.	☐	☐	☐	_____
3. Adjust the bed to a comfortable height.	☐	☐	☐	_____
4. Lower the client's head to as flat a position as he or she can tolerate, and lower the side rail.	☐	☐	☐	_____
5. Move the client to the side of the bed. Raise the side rail.	☐	☐	☐	_____
6. Have the client reach for the side rail.	☐	☐	☐	_____
7. Assume a broad stance, tensing abdominal and gluteal muscles. Roll the client toward you.	☐	☐	☐	_____
8. Position the client's legs comfortably:	☐	☐	☐	_____
a. Flex his or her lower knee and hip slightly.	☐	☐	☐	_____
b. Bring his or her upper leg forward, and place a pillow between the legs.	☐	☐	☐	_____
9. Adjust the client's arms:	☐	☐	☐	_____
a. Shift his or her lower shoulder slightly toward you.	☐	☐	☐	_____
b. Support his or her upper arm on a pillow.	☐	☐	☐	_____
10. Wedge a pillow behind the client's back. Use rolled blankets or towels as needed for support.	☐	☐	☐	_____
11. Lower the bed, elevate the head of the bed as the client can tolerate, and raise the side rail.	☐	☐	☐	_____
12. Wash hands.	☐	☐	☐	_____

KEY: E = Excels   S = Satisfactory   NP = Needs Practice

☐ **Pass**   ☐ **Fail**

Student's Signature: _____ Date: _____

Instructor's Signature: _____ Date: _____

Performing PROM Exercises

RECOMMENDED TECHNIQUE	E	S	NP	Comments
1. Wash hands.	☐	☐	☐	_____
2. Explain the procedure to the client.	☐	☐	☐	_____
3. Adjust the bed to a comfortable height. Select one side of the bed to begin PROM exercises.	☐	☐	☐	_____
4. Uncover only the limb to be exercised.	☐	☐	☐	_____
5. Support all joints during exercise activity.	☐	☐	☐	_____
6. Use slow, gentle movements when performing exercises. Repeat each exercise three times. Stop if the client complains of pain or discomfort.	☐	☐	☐	_____
7. Begin exercises with the client's neck and work downward.	☐	☐	☐	_____
8. Flex, extend, and rotate the client's neck. Support his or her head with your hands.	☐	☐	☐	_____
9. Exercise the client's shoulder and elbow:	☐	☐	☐	_____
a. Support the client's elbow with one hand, and grasp the client's wrist with other hand.	☐	☐	☐	_____
b. Raise the client's arm from the side to above the head.	☐	☐	☐	_____
c. Perform internal rotation by moving the client's arm across his or her chest.	☐	☐	☐	_____
d. Externally rotate the client's shoulder by moving the arm away from the client.	☐	☐	☐	_____
e. Flex and extend the client's elbow.	☐	☐	☐	_____
10. Perform all exercises on the client's wrist and fingers:	☐	☐	☐	_____
a. Flex and extend the wrist.	☐	☐	☐	_____
b. Abduct and adduct the wrist.	☐	☐	☐	_____
c. Flex and extend the client's fingers.	☐	☐	☐	_____
d. Abduct and adduct the fingers.	☐	☐	☐	_____
e. Rotate the thumb.	☐	☐	☐	_____
11. Exercise the client's hip and leg:	☐	☐	☐	_____
a. Flex and extend the hip and knee while supporting the leg.	☐	☐	☐	_____
b. Abduct and adduct the hip by moving the client's straightened leg and then back to median position.	☐	☐	☐	_____

RECOMMENDED TECHNIQUE (*Continued*)	E	S	NP	Comments
c. Perform internal and external rotation of the hip joint by turning the leg inward and then outward.	☐	☐	☐	_____
12. Perform exercises on the ankle and foot:	☐	☐	☐	_____
a. Dorsiflex and plantar flex the foot.	☐	☐	☐	_____
b. Abduct and adduct the toes.	☐	☐	☐	_____
c. Evert and invert the foot.	☐	☐	☐	_____
13. Move to the other side of the bed and repeat exercises.	☐	☐	☐	_____
14. Reposition and cover the client. Return the bed to low position.	☐	☐	☐	_____
15. Wash hands.	☐	☐	☐	_____
16. Document completion of PROM exercises.	☐	☐	☐	_____

KEY: E = Excels   S = Satisfactory   NP = Needs Practice

☐ **Pass**   ☐ **Fail**

Student's Signature: _____ Date: _____

Instructor's Signature: _____ Date: _____

Helping the Client Into a Wheelchair or Chair

SUPPLIES AND EQUIPMENT
✔ Wheelchair
✔ Slippers or shoes (non-skid soles)
✔ Robe
✔ Transfer belt (optional)

RECOMMENDED TECHNIQUE	E	S	NP	Comments
1. Wash hands.	☐	☐	☐	_____
2. Explain the procedure to the client.	☐	☐	☐	_____
3. Position the wheelchair next to the bed or at a 45-degree angle to the bed. Lock the wheel brakes and remove the foot rests or move them to the "up" position.	☐	☐	☐	_____
4. Prepare to move the client:	☐	☐	☐	_____
a. Assist the client with putting on robe and slippers.	☐	☐	☐	_____
b. Obtain help from another person if the client is immobile, heavy, or connected to multiple pieces of equipment.	☐	☐	☐	_____
5. Raise the head of the bed so that the client is in the sitting position.	☐	☐	☐	_____
6. Assist the client to sit on the side of the bed:	☐	☐	☐	_____
a. Support the head and neck with one arm.	☐	☐	☐	_____
b. Use other arm to move the client's leg over the side of the bed.	☐	☐	☐	_____
c. Allow the client's feet to rest on the floor.	☐	☐	☐	_____
d. Maintain the client in this position for a short time.	☐	☐	☐	_____
7. Prepare to raise the client to a standing position:	☐	☐	☐	_____
a. Apply a transfer belt if necessary.	☐	☐	☐	_____
b. Spread the client's feet and brace your knees against the client's knees.	☐	☐	☐	_____
c. Place your arms around the client's waist.	☐	☐	☐	_____
8. Use a rocking motion of the legs to assist the client to stand. The client may use his or her hands to help push upward from bed.	☐	☐	☐	_____

RECOMMENDED TECHNIQUE (*Continued*)	E	S	NP	Comments
9. Pivot the client into position immediately in front of the wheelchair. Encourage the client to use arm rests for support while lowering into chair.	☐	☐	☐	_____
10. Reposition foot rests. Secure the client in a chair with a safety belt if needed. Cover the client with a blanket. Provide the nurse call button.	☐	☐	☐	_____
11. Wash hands.	☐	☐	☐	_____
12. Check on the client frequently.	☐	☐	☐	_____
13. Document the transfer and the client's response.	☐	☐	☐	_____

KEY: E = Excels   S = Satisfactory   NP = Needs Practice

☐ **Pass**   ☐ **Fail**

Student's Signature: _____ Date: _____

Instructor's Signature: _____ Date: _____

Assisting the Immobile Client to Move Up in Bed

SUPPLIES AND EQUIPMENT
✔ Pillows
✔ Side rails
✔ Overhead trapeze (optional)
✔ Draw sheet (optional)

RECOMMENDED TECHNIQUE	E	S	NP	Comments
1. Wash hands.	☐	☐	☐	_____
2. Explain the procedure to the client.	☐	☐	☐	_____
3. Adjust the bed to a comfortable height.	☐	☐	☐	_____
4. Lower the bed to as flat a position as the client can tolerate, and lower the side rail.	☐	☐	☐	_____
5. Lock the wheels on the bed.	☐	☐	☐	_____
6. Remove the pillow from under the client's head, and place it against the head of the bed.	☐	☐	☐	_____
7. Assist the client to flex the knees and hips with feet flat on the bed.	☐	☐	☐	_____
8. Ask the client to assist with the move by:				
a. Folding his or her arms across the chest.	☐	☐	☐	_____
b. Using an overhead trapeze (if available) to lift and pull the body upward.	☐	☐	☐	_____
c. Pushing upward with the feet.	☐	☐	☐	_____
d. Grasping the top of the bed and pulling with both hands.	☐	☐	☐	_____
9. Assume a broad-based stance by flexing knees and hips with feet spread and turned toward the head of the bed.	☐	☐	☐	_____
10. Slide arms under the client's shoulders and thighs.	☐	☐	☐	_____
11. Rock weight onto back leg and shift upward with the client's assistance on the count of three. Repeat steps if necessary to advance the client further up in bed.	☐	☐	☐	_____
12. Replace the pillow under the client's head. Lower the bed and elevate the head as the client can tolerate. Raise side rail.	☐	☐	☐	_____
13. Wash hands.	☐	☐	☐	_____

KEY: E = Excels   S = Satisfactory   NP = Needs Practice

☐ **Pass**   ☐ **Fail**

Student's Signature: _____ Date: _____

Instructor's Signature: _____ Date: _____

Making an Unoccupied Bed

SUPPLIES AND EQUIPMENT
✔ Gloves (optional)
✔ Two sheets (either two flat sheets or one flat sheet and one contour bottom sheet)
✔ Draw sheet (optional)
✔ Blanket
✔ Bedspread
✔ Pillowcases
✔ Linen hamper or bag
✔ Mattress pad
✔ Bedside table or chair

RECOMMENDED TECHNIQUE	E	S	NP	Comments
1. Gather linens and supplies.	☐	☐	☐	_____
2. Wash hands.	☐	☐	☐	_____
3. Adjust the bed to a comfortable height. Remove the call bell if it is attached.	☐	☐	☐	_____
4. Wear gloves if the linens are soiled. Loosen all soiled linens. Remove, roll up, and place them in a linen hamper or bag. Never place soiled linens on the floor or hold them against your uniform.	☐	☐	☐	_____
5. Refold the spread or any item that is to be reused. Place it on the table or the back of the chair.	☐	☐	☐	_____
6. Remove soiled pillowcases and place them in the linen hamper. Move pillows to the chair.	☐	☐	☐	_____
7. Slide the mattress to the head of the bed. Place a mattress pad on the bed.	☐	☐	☐	_____
8. Place a bottom sheet on the bed. Open it lengthwise with the centerfold along the bed's center. Fold back the upper layer of the sheet toward the opposite side of the bed. Slide the sheet upward over the top of the bed, leaving the bottom edge of the sheet even with the edge of the mattress. If using a fitted (contour) sheet, tuck it over the mattress at the upper and lower end of that side.	☐	☐	☐	_____
9. Tuck the sheet securely under the head of the mattress. Make a diagonal or mitered corner (45-degree angle) if the sheet is not fitted:	☐	☐	☐	_____
a. Pick up the selvage edge with the hand nearest the foot of the bed.	☐	☐	☐	_____
b. Lay a triangle back on the bed.	☐	☐	☐	_____
c. Tuck the hanging part of the sheet under the mattress.	☐	☐	☐	_____
d. Drop the triangle over the side of the bed.	☐	☐	☐	_____
e. Tuck the hanging edge under the mattress.	☐	☐	☐	_____

RECOMMENDED TECHNIQUE (*Continued*)	E	S	NP	Comments

10. Tuck the sheet under the entire side of bed. ☐ ☐ ☐ _____

11. Place a draw sheet on the bed (if used), folded in half, with the fold in the center of the bed. Lift the top half backward toward the other side of the bed. Tuck the draw sheet under the mattress. ☐ ☐ ☐ _____

12. Place the top sheet on the bed, centering it in the same manner as the bottom sheet. Make sure the upper hem of the top sheet is level with the top of the mattress. Drop the lower end of the sheet over the end of the mattress. ☐ ☐ ☐ _____

13. Cover the top sheet with a blanket or bed-spread. Tuck all these together under the bottom of the mattress. Miter the corner. ☐ ☐ ☐ _____

14. Move to the other side of the bed. Tuck in the bottom linens as in step 13. Fold back the cuff at the head of the bed with the sheet and bedspread if the client will be returning to bed. (Pull linens up to the top of the bed when making a closed bed.) ☐ ☐ ☐ _____

15. Put a clean pillow case on the pillow: ☐ ☐ ☐ _____

   a. Rest the pillow on a flat surface. ☐ ☐ ☐ _____

   b. Grasp the pillow case in the center on the closed end. ☐ ☐ ☐ _____

   c. Turn the pillowcase back over the hand. ☐ ☐ ☐ _____

   d. Grasp the pillow through the pillow case. ☐ ☐ ☐ _____

   e. Pull the pillow case over the pillow. ☐ ☐ ☐ _____

   f. Adjust the pillow case smoothly over the pillow. An alternate method is to put one hand inside the pillow case and pull the pillow corners into the corners of the pillow case. ☐ ☐ ☐ _____

16. Place a pillow at the top of the bed in the center with the open end away from the door. ☐ ☐ ☐ _____

17. Make a toe pleat at the foot of the bed: ☐ ☐ ☐ _____

   a. For a horizontal pleat, gather the linens to make a fold approximately 5 to 10 cm (2–4 inches) across the foot of the bed. ☐ ☐ ☐ _____

   b. For a vertical pleat, gather the linens to make a fold approximately 5 to 10 cm (2–4 inches) perpendicular (up and down) to the foot of the bed. ☐ ☐ ☐ _____

RECOMMENDED TECHNIQUE (*Continued*)	E	S	NP	Comments
18. Fanfold the top of the linens to the bottom third of the bed. This is called an open bed.	☐	☐	☐	_____
19. Replace the call signal on the bed, and secure it in place.	☐	☐	☐	_____
20. Move the overbed table next to the bed.	☐	☐	☐	_____
21. Return the bed to low position if the client is ambulatory or high position if the client is returning to the room by stretcher.	☐	☐	☐	_____
22. Discard linens appropriately. Wash hands.	☐	☐	☐	_____

KEY: E = Excels   S = Satisfactory   NP = Needs Practice

☐ **Pass**   ☐ **Fail**

Student's Signature: _____ Date: _____

Instructor's Signature: _____ Date: _____

Making an Occupied Bed

SUPPLIES AND EQUIPMENT

✔ Gloves (optional)
✔ Two sheets (either two flat sheets or one flat sheet and one contour bottom sheet)
✔ Draw sheet (optional)
✔ Blanket
✔ Bedspread

✔ Pillowcases
✔ Linen hamper or bag
✔ Mattress pad
✔ Bedside table or chair
✔ Bath blanket (optional)

RECOMMENDED TECHNIQUE	E	S	NP	Comments
1. Gather linens and supplies.	☐	☐	☐	_____
2. Explain the procedure to the client.	☐	☐	☐	_____
3. Wash hands prior to putting on gloves.	☐	☐	☐	_____
4. Adjust the bed to a comfortable height. Remove the call bell if it is attached to linens. Lower the side rail on the near side, while keeping the other side rail raised.	☐	☐	☐	_____
5. Lower the head of the bed if the client can tolerate it.	☐	☐	☐	_____
6. Loosen the top bed linens. Remove the spread. Refold it if it will be reused, and place it on the table or back of the chair.	☐	☐	☐	_____
7. Place a bath blanket over the top sheet. Remove the top sheet and place it in the linen hamper or bag. If a bath blanket is unavailable, leave the top sheet in place.	☐	☐	☐	_____
8. Slide the mattress to the head of the bed if necessary. Request assistance to do this.	☐	☐	☐	_____
9. Assist the client to turn toward the other side of the bed. Adjust the pillow. The client can help by hanging onto the side rail, if able.	☐	☐	☐	_____
10. Loosen bottom bed linens. Fanfold soiled linens from the side of the bed and wedge them close to the client. Leave the mattress pad in place unless soiled.	☐	☐	☐	_____
11. Place the clean bottom sheet on the bed folded lengthwise with the centerfold as close to the client's back as possible. Adjust the sheet, miter the upper corner, and place the draw sheet (optional). If using the fitted (contour) sheet, tuck it over the mattress at the upper and lower ends. Fold upper half of the sheet and draw it back toward the center. Tuck it under the client and under soiled linens.	☐	☐	☐	_____

RECOMMENDED TECHNIQUE (*Continued*)	E	S	NP	Comments
12. Raise the side rail. Move to the bed's other side. Help the client roll over the folded linen to the other side of the bed. Lower the side rail. Readjust the pillow and bath blanket.	☐	☐	☐	_____
13. Remove the soiled bottom linens. Hold them away from clothing. Place them in the hamper or bag. Straighten the mattress pad.	☐	☐	☐	_____
14. Grasp clean linens and gently pull them out from under the client. Spread them over the bed's unmade side. Pull the linens taut and tuck in the bottom sheet. Miter the corner. If using a contour sheet, tuck it in both the top and bottom corners. Brace knee against the bed. Pull the bottom sheet and draw sheet taut prior to tucking them under the mattress.	☐	☐	☐	_____
15. Assist the client back to the center of the bed. Remove the pillow. Replace the soiled pillow case with a clean one, and return the pillow to the bed under the client's head.	☐	☐	☐	_____
16. Place the top sheet over the bath blanket. Ask the client to hold onto the upper edge. Remove the bath blanket and place it in the linen hamper, bag, or client's closet. Unfold the spread over the top sheet. Tuck the lower ends securely under mattress. Miter corners.	☐	☐	☐	_____
17. Turn the top edge of the spread back over the sheet.	☐	☐	☐	_____
18. Make a toe pleat or loosen the top linens over the client's feet.	☐	☐	☐	_____
19. Raise side rail. Lower the bed and adjust the head to a comfortable position. Replace the call signal on the bed.	☐	☐	☐	_____
20. Discard linens appropriately. Remove gloves and wash hands.	☐	☐	☐	_____

KEY: E = Excels   S = Satisfactory   NP = Needs Practice

☐ **Pass**   ☐ **Fail**

Student's Signature: _____ Date: _____

Instructor's Signature: _____ Date: _____

Giving Special Mouth Care

SUPPLIES AND EQUIPMENT
- ✔ Gloves
- ✔ Toothbrush or sponge toothette
- ✔ Tongue blade padded with a 4 × 4 gauze sponge
- ✔ Water, mouthwash, or hydrogen peroxide (H_2O_2)
- ✔ Towel
- ✔ Water-soluble lubricant for lips
- ✔ Suction catheter with suction apparatus (optional)
- ✔ Emesis basin

RECOMMENDED TECHNIQUE	E	S	NP	Comments
1. Gather supplies.	☐	☐	☐	_____
2. Explain the procedure to the client.	☐	☐	☐	_____
3. Wash hands and put on gloves.	☐	☐	☐	_____
4. Close the curtain or door to the room.	☐	☐	☐	_____
5. Raise the bed to a comfortable height. Lower the near side rail. Turn the client on the side with the head tilted down toward the mattress.	☐	☐	☐	_____
6. Place a towel and emesis basin under the client's chin. Have a suction catheter and apparatus available if needed.	☐	☐	☐	_____
7. Open the client's mouth and insert the padded tongue blade toward the back molar area. Never insert fingers into the client's mouth.	☐	☐	☐	_____
8. Dip a toothette sponge, soft toothbrush, or another padded tongue blade in water, mouthwash, or diluted H_2O_2. Move it back and forth gently across the client's teeth and chewing areas. Cleanse the roof of the mouth and the inner cheek area.	☐	☐	☐	_____
9. Rinse the areas using a clean toothette or padded tongue blade in moistened water. Suction any drainage if necessary.	☐	☐	☐	_____
10. Apply water-soluble lubricant to the client's lips.	☐	☐	☐	_____
11. Reposition the client. Lower the bed and raise the side rail.	☐	☐	☐	_____
12. Remove gloves and wash hands.	☐	☐	☐	_____
13. Document assessments on the health record.	☐	☐	☐	_____

KEY: E = Excels   S = Satisfactory   NP = Needs Practice

☐ **Pass**   ☐ **Fail**

Student's Signature: _____ Date: _____

Instructor's Signature: _____ Date: _____

Shaving a Client

SUPPLIES AND EQUIPMENT

✔ Razor: safety or electric
✔ Wash basin
✔ Warm water
✔ Disposable gloves

✔ Shaving cream or soap
✔ Aftershave lotion, if desired
✔ Moisturizer
✔ Towels

(Some of these supplies may not be needed if an electric razor is used.)

RECOMMENDED TECHNIQUE	E	S	NP	Comments
1. Explain the procedure to the client.	☐	☐	☐	_____
2. Place the client in a position that is comfortable for both the client and nurse.	☐	☐	☐	_____
3. Put on gloves.	☐	☐	☐	_____
4. Place a warm, wet washcloth on the area to be shaved for a few seconds.	☐	☐	☐	_____
5. Apply shaving cream or soap to the area if using a blade razor.	☐	☐	☐	_____
6. Hold the skin taut while making strokes.	☐	☐	☐	_____
7. Holding the blade razor at a 45-degree angle to the skin, move it across the skin in short strokes in the direction the hair grows. If using an electric razor, move it across the area as needed until the entire beard is cut.	☐	☐	☐	_____
8. Wash the shaven area thoroughly with a clean, warm, moistened washcloth.	☐	☐	☐	_____
9. Pat the area dry.	☐	☐	☐	_____
10. For men, apply aftershave lotion if the client prefers.	☐	☐	☐	_____
11. If shaving a woman's legs or underarms, apply moisturizer if the client prefers.	☐	☐	☐	_____
12. If a disposable blade razor is used, discard it in the sharps container; if using the client's own razor, cover the blade, and store it in a safe place to prevent cuts and loss.	☐	☐	☐	_____
a. Clean the client's electric razor thoroughly after each use by removing the faceplate and blades and cleaning the blades and surrounding areas with the small brush provided or a disposable toothbrush. Brush out all beard stubble and skin debris.	☐	☐	☐	_____

RECOMMENDED TECHNIQUE (*Continued*)	E	S	NP	Comments
b. Clean all surfaces around the blades with an alcohol wipe, and allow to dry before reassembling.	☐	☐	☐	_____
c. Plug in the razor for recharging if necessary.	☐	☐	☐	_____
13. Properly dispose of gloves.	☐	☐	☐	_____
14. Document the procedure in the client's record.	☐	☐	☐	_____

KEY: E = Excels   S = Satisfactory   NP = Needs Practice

☐ **Pass**   ☐ **Fail**

Student's Signature: _____   Date: _____

Instructor's Signature: _____   Date: _____

Shampooing a Client's Hair in Bed

SUPPLIES AND EQUIPMENT
✔ Comb or hair pick and brush
✔ One bath towel, two hand towels, one washcloth
✔ Plastic for floor and chair
✔ One large pitcher of water
✔ Cotton balls
✔ One small pitcher for pouring

✔ Shampoo or mild soap solution
✔ One pail
✔ Shampoo trough
✔ Moisture-proof pillowcase
✔ Gloves
✔ Conditioner and hair dryer (optional)

RECOMMENDED TECHNIQUE	E	S	NP	Comments
1. Check to ensure that a physician's order is on the client's health record.	☐	☐	☐	_____
2. Wash hands and put on gloves.	☐	☐	☐	_____
3. Cover the client with a bath blanket and turn back the bedcovers.	☐	☐	☐	_____
4. Cover the pillow with a moisture-proof case and place it under the client's head.	☐	☐	☐	_____
5. Raise the bed to the highest position, and place the head of the bed in the flat position.	☐	☐	☐	_____
6. Gently move the client's head and shoulders to the edge of the bed nearest the nurse.	☐	☐	☐	_____
7. Comb and brush the client's hair thoroughly.	☐	☐	☐	_____
8. Place plastic on the floor.	☐	☐	☐	_____
9. Place the pail on a covered chair.	☐	☐	☐	_____
10. Place the shampoo basin under the client's head with the trough directed to the side of the bed so that water flows into the pail.	☐	☐	☐	_____
11. Cover the client with an extra bath blanket.	☐	☐	☐	_____
12. Secure a folded towel around the client's neck.	☐	☐	☐	_____
13. Cover the client's eyes with a damp wash cloth, and place cotton in his or her ears.	☐	☐	☐	_____
14. Place a towel over the client's chest.	☐	☐	☐	_____
15. Wet hair thoroughly with warm water (about 105° to 110°F, 40.6° to 42°C).	☐	☐	☐	_____
16. Apply shampoo or mild soap solution, using enough to make a thick lather, and rub it into and massage the scalp as you do so.	☐	☐	☐	_____
17. Rinse well.	☐	☐	☐	_____
18. Reapply shampoo, massage, and rinse thoroughly.	☐	☐	☐	_____

RECOMMENDED TECHNIQUE (*Continued*)	E	S	NP	Comments
19. Apply conditioner and rinse.	☐	☐	☐	_____
20. Squeeze excess water from the hair and wrap a towel around the client's head. Gently pat or rub to dry hair. Wrap a dry towel around the client's damp hair.	☐	☐	☐	_____
21. Remove wet towels and equipment.	☐	☐	☐	_____
22. Use a hair dryer, comb or hair pick, and brush as needed.	☐	☐	☐	_____
23. Dispose of gloves, and wash your hands.	☐	☐	☐	_____
24. Document the procedure, and note how the client tolerated it.	☐	☐	☐	_____

KEY: E = Excels   S = Satisfactory   NP = Needs Practice

☐ **Pass**   ☐ **Fail**

Student's Signature: _____   Date: _____

Instructor's Signature: _____   Date: _____

Giving Perineal Care

SUPPLIES AND EQUIPMENT
✔ Gloves
✔ Wash cloths
✔ Basin
✔ Waterproof pad

✔ Towels
✔ Soap
✔ Toilet tissue
✔ Bath blanket

RECOMMENDED TECHNIQUE	E	S	NP	Comments
1. Gather supplies.	☐	☐	☐	_____
2. Explain the procedure to the client.	☐	☐	☐	_____
3. Wash hands and put on gloves.	☐	☐	☐	_____
4. Close the curtain or the door to the room.	☐	☐	☐	_____
5. Raise the bed to a comfortable height. Lower the near side rail.	☐	☐	☐	_____
6. Uncover the client's perineal area. Place a towel or waterproof pad under the client's hips.	☐	☐	☐	_____
7. Make a mitt with the washcloth. Cleanse the client's upper thighs and groin area with soap and water. Rinse and dry. Wash the genital area next.				
Female Client				
a. Use a separate portion of the washcloth for each stroke, changing washcloths as necessary.	☐	☐	☐	_____
b. Separate the labia and cleanse downward from the pubic to anal area.	☐	☐	☐	_____
c. Wash between the labia, including the urethral meatus and vaginal area. Rinse well and pat dry.				
Male Client				
a. Gently grasp the client's penis.	☐	☐	☐	_____
b. Cleanse in a circular motion moving from the tip of the penis downward toward the pubic area.	☐	☐	☐	_____
c. Retract the foreskin in an uncircumcised male prior to washing the penis.	☐	☐	☐	_____
d. Rinse well and dry.	☐	☐	☐	_____
e. Return the foreskin to its former position.	☐	☐	☐	_____
f. Wash, rinse, and dry the perineum and scrotum carefully.	☐	☐	☐	_____
8. Assist the client to turn on the side. Separate the client's buttocks, and use toilet tissue, if necessary, to remove fecal material.	☐	☐	☐	_____

RECOMMENDED TECHNIQUE (*Continued*)   **E   S   NP   Comments**

9. Cleanse the anal area, rinse thoroughly, and dry with a towel. (In some cases, shaving cream is more effective and comfortable to use than soap when cleaning the anal area.) Change washcloths as necessary.   ☐   ☐   ☐   _____

10. Apply skin care products to the area according to need or physician's order.   ☐   ☐   ☐   _____

11. Return the client to a comfortable position. Lower the bed, and raise the side rail as ordered.   ☐   ☐   ☐   _____

12. Remove gloves and wash your hands.   ☐   ☐   ☐   _____

13. Document the procedure, describing the client's skin condition.   ☐   ☐   ☐   _____

KEY: E = Excels   S = Satisfactory   NP = Needs Practice

☐ **Pass**   ☐ **Fail**

Student's Signature: _____   Date: _____

Instructor's Signature: _____   Date: _____

Giving a Bed Bath

SUPPLIES AND EQUIPMENT
- ✔ Gloves (optional)
- ✔ Bath blanket
- ✔ Towels
- ✔ Washcloths
- ✔ Basin
- ✔ Gown or pajamas
- ✔ Personal items (e.g., deodorant, powder)
- ✔ Bedpan or urinal
- ✔ Clean bed linens
- ✔ Linen hamper or bag
- ✔ Soap

RECOMMENDED TECHNIQUE	E	S	NP	Comments
1. Gather supplies.	☐	☐	☐	_____
2. Explain the procedure to the client. If he or she is alert and oriented, question the client about personal hygiene preferences and ability to assist with the bath.	☐	☐	☐	_____
3. Wash hands and put on gloves.	☐	☐	☐	_____
4. Close the curtain or the door.	☐	☐	☐	_____
5. Provide the client with an opportunity to use a bedpan or urinal.	☐	☐	☐	_____
6. Raise the bed to a comfortable working height.	☐	☐	☐	_____
7. Remove the bedspread, fold it, and place it on a chair or table. Cover the client with a bath blanket. Remove the top sheet while the client holds onto the bath blanket.	☐	☐	☐	_____
8. Fill the basin about two-thirds full with warm water (110° to 115°F [43° to 46°C]), and place it on the bedside table.	☐	☐	☐	_____
9. Lower the near side rail if it is raised. Remove the client's gown, and keep the bath blanket in place, covering the client. If an IV catheter is present on the client's upper extremity, thread the IV tubing and bag through the sleeve of the soiled gown. Rehang the IV solution. Check the IV flow rate or pump activity.	☐	☐	☐	_____
10. Assist the client to move toward the side of the bed nearest the nurse. Usually the nurse will complete most of the work with the dominant hand.	☐	☐	☐	_____
11. Make a mitt with the washcloth by holding the top two corners so the washcloth is around the back of the hand, with the open side across the palm. Then tuck the loose end into the top, enclosing the fingers.	☐	☐	☐	_____

RECOMMENDED TECHNIQUE (*Continued*)	E	S	NP	Comments
12. Moisten the mitt with plain water, and wash the client's eyes. Cleanse from the inner corner (near nose) to the outer corner of each eye. Use a different section of the mitt to wash each eye.	☐	☐	☐	_____
13. Wash the client's face, neck, and ears. Use soap on these areas only if the client prefers. Dry these areas carefully.	☐	☐	☐	_____
14. Uncover the client's far arm. Place a bath towel under it. Wash with long strokes, rinse, and dry the area. Pay special attention to the axilla.	☐	☐	☐	_____
15. Place the basin on a folded towel. Immerse the client's opposite hand in the water. Wash, rinse, and dry. Cover the client's arm with the bath blanket. Repeat these steps for the client's near arm and hand.	☐	☐	☐	_____
16. Open a bath towel over the client's chest, and fold the bath blanket back. Wash, rinse, and dry the client's chest. Wash, assess, and carefully dry the skin under the female client's breasts. Apply powder if the client desires.	☐	☐	☐	_____
17. Keep the towel over the client's chest, and lower the bath blanket to just above the pubic area. Wash, rinse, and dry the abdomen, paying special attention to the umbilicus or any skin folds. Cover the client's chest and abdomen with the bath blanket, and remove the towel. The client may put a gown on at this time, leaving it untied at the neck.	☐	☐	☐	_____
18. Uncover the client's far leg, and place a towel under it. Wash with long strokes; rinse and dry the leg.	☐	☐	☐	_____
19. Place the basin on a folded bath towel, and carefully immerse the client's far foot in water. Wash, rinse, and dry the foot, paying particular attention to the area between the toes. Cover the leg and foot with the bath blanket. Repeat on the other side.	☐	☐	☐	_____
20. Raise the side rail, and change bath water at this point.	☐	☐	☐	_____
21. Lower the near side rail. Assist the client to turn away from you onto his or her side. Uncover the client's back and buttocks. Place an opened towel on the bed parallel to the client's back. Wash, rinse,				

RECOMMENDED TECHNIQUE (*Continued*)	E	S	NP	Comments
and dry the client's back and buttocks. Wash the rectal area. Assess for reddened areas or any skin breakdown.	☐	☐	☐	_____
22. Give a backrub at this time. Tie or snap the client's gown at the back or side of the neck.	☐	☐	☐	_____
23. Return the client to his or her back, and adjust the bath blanket so that the client is covered. Use side rails for safety, and change bath water again. Use a clean washcloth and towel to wash the client's perineal area (if the client is unable). Otherwise, place necessary equipment within the client's reach, and allow him or her to complete this care. Provide privacy. Cover the client with the bath blanket. Remove gloves and discard them in the proper receptacle.	☐	☐	☐	_____
24. Help the client put on a gown or pajamas (if this was not done before). Assist the client with personal hygiene, such as deodorant and cologne. Assist with hair care and oral hygiene.	☐	☐	☐	_____
25. Make the bed with clean linens. Lower the bed and raise the side rails as ordered.	☐	☐	☐	_____
26. Wash hands.	☐	☐	☐	_____
27. Document assessments on flow sheet and chart.	☐	☐	☐	_____

KEY: E = Excels   S = Satisfactory   NP = Needs Practice

☐ **Pass**   ☐ **Fail**

Student's Signature: _____ Date: _____

Instructor's Signature: _____ Date: _____

Giving and Removing the Bedpan

SUPPLIES AND EQUIPMENT
- ✔ Gloves
- ✔ Cover for bedpan
- ✔ Handwashing supplies
- ✔ Bedpan
- ✔ Toilet tissue
- ✔ Air freshener (optional)

RECOMMENDED TECHNIQUE	E	S	NP	Comments
1. Obtain a bedpan if one is not available in the bedside cabinet.	☐	☐	☐	_____
2. Explain the procedure to the client.	☐	☐	☐	_____
3. Wash hands and put on gloves.	☐	☐	☐	_____
4. Close the curtain or door to the room.	☐	☐	☐	_____
5. Raise the bed to a comfortable height. Lower the near side rail.	☐	☐	☐	_____
6. Fold the bed linen away from the client, exposing as little of his or her body as possible. Place an incontinence pad on the bed if the client is confused or if using a fracture pan.	☐	☐	☐	_____
7. Assist the client onto the bedpan. If the client is able to help, encourage him or her to flex the knees and lift the hips.	☐	☐	☐	_____
a. Place the bedpan under the buttocks with the rounded curved end toward the client's back and the narrower, open end toward the feet.	☐	☐	☐	_____
b. If a client is unable to use a regular bedpan, use a fracture bedpan. Place it under the buttocks with the flat end toward the client's back.	☐	☐	☐	_____
8. If the client is immobile, roll the client onto his or her side away from you. Position the bedpan against the client's buttocks, hold it firmly in place, and turn the client onto his or her back. Check the pan's location.	☐	☐	☐	_____
9. Replace the bed linen over the client.	☐	☐	☐	_____
10. Elevate the head of the bed to semi-Fowler's position if the client can tolerate it. Raise the side rail again.	☐	☐	☐	_____
11. Place the call light and toilet tissue within the client's reach, and leave him or her alone if possible. Tell the client to call if he or she needs help and when finished. If leaving the bedside, remove gloves, and wash hands.	☐	☐	☐	_____

RECOMMENDED TECHNIQUE (*Continued*)	E	S	NP	Comments
12. To remove the bedpan:	☐	☐	☐	_____
a. Wash hands and put on gloves.	☐	☐	☐	_____
b. Lower the side rail and the head of the bed.	☐	☐	☐	_____
c. Uncover the client.	☐	☐	☐	_____
d. Fold the toilet tissue and wipe from the front (pubic area) to the back (anus) if the client is unable to do so independently.	☐	☐	☐	_____
e. Steady the bedpan as the client either lifts the hips or is assisted to turn away from you.	☐	☐	☐	_____
f. Place the bedpan on the chair and cover it.	☐	☐	☐	_____
g. Cleanse the area with soap and water if necessary. Shaving lather works well and is soothing. Dry carefully.	☐	☐	☐	_____
13. Offer handwashing supplies to the client.	☐	☐	☐	_____
14. Return the client to a comfortable position. Lower the bed, and raise the side rail. Use air freshener if necessary.	☐	☐	☐	_____
15. Empty the pan into the toilet and rinse. Measure output or obtain stool sample if ordered. Remove gloves and wash hands.	☐	☐	☐	_____
16. Document results according to agency policy on flow sheet, intake and output summary, or chart.	☐	☐	☐	_____

Emptying the Drainage Bag

SUPPLIES AND EQUIPMENT
✔ Disposable gloves
✔ Measuring container or graduated container

RECOMMENDED TECHNIQUE	E	S	NP	Comments
1. Wash hands and put on clean gloves.	☐	☐	☐	_____
2. Carefully pull the drain tube (located on the bottom of the bag) out of the storage pocket without touching it below the level of the clamp.	☐	☐	☐	_____
3. Hold the tube over the container and release the clamp, making sure that the drain tube does not touch anything.	☐	☐	☐	_____
4. When the urine has drained out, clamp the tube, and carefully replace it into the storage pocket. Be sure the clamp is far enough up the tube to allow most of the tube to fit into the pocket. Do not move the clamp up on the tube.	☐	☐	☐	_____
5. Collect the urine in a graduated container and measure it.	☐	☐	☐	_____
6. Observe the color, odor, and other characteristics of urine.	☐	☐	☐	_____
7. Discard urine (unless a specimen is required), and rinse the graduated container with cool water.	☐	☐	☐	_____
8. Explain each step of emptying the drainage bag to the client and family if the client will be discharged from the health care agency with the catheter.	☐	☐	☐	_____
9. Ask the client or a family member to do a return demonstration after you have demonstrated the procedure.	☐	☐	☐	_____
10. Remove and discard gloves and wash hands.	☐	☐	☐	_____
11. Record output on the appropriate sheet, and document and report any special observations about the urine.	☐	☐	☐	_____

KEY: E = Excels   S = Satisfactory   NP = Needs Practice

☐ **Pass**   ☐ **Fail**

Student's Signature: _____ Date: _____

Instructor's Signature: _____ Date: _____

Giving a Cleansing Enema: Can (Bucket)-and-Tubing Method

SUPPLIES AND EQUIPMENT

- ✔ Gloves
- ✔ Disposable enema setup, including container, tubing, and clamp (approximate rectal tube size: adult 22–0 Fr, child 12–18 Fr)
- ✔ Solution as prescribed
- ✔ Bedpan and cover

- ✔ Toilet tissue
- ✔ Waterproof pad
- ✔ Water-soluble lubricant
- ✔ Bath blanket
- ✔ Cleansing supplies
- ✔ IV pole

RECOMMENDED TECHNIQUE	E	S	NP	Comments
1. Gather supplies. Use a latex-free tube if the client is allergic to latex.	☐	☐	☐	_____
2. Explain the procedure to the client.	☐	☐	☐	_____
3. Wash hands and put on gloves.	☐	☐	☐	_____
4. Prepare the enema:	☐	☐	☐	_____
a. Fill the enema can with prescribed solution at proper temperature (adults, 100° to 110°F; children, 100°F).	☐	☐	☐	_____
b. Open the clamp, and allow fluid to flow through the tubing.	☐	☐	☐	_____
c. Reclamp the tubing.	☐	☐	☐	_____
5. Close the curtain or door to the room.	☐	☐	☐	_____
6. Raise the bed to a comfortable working height. Lower the near side rail.	☐	☐	☐	_____
7. Place a waterproof pad under the client's buttocks.	☐	☐	☐	_____
8. Assist the client to turn onto the left side with the right knee flexed. Place a bedpan in bed close to the client. If the client is unable to retain the enema solution, place him or her on the bedpan (some clients will be able to go into the bathroom to expel the solution).	☐	☐	☐	_____
9. Lubricate the tip of the rectal tube 2 to 3 inches (if it is not prelubricated).	☐	☐	☐	_____
10. Place the enema can on an IV pole or raise the container approximately 18 inches above the client's anus.	☐	☐	☐	_____
11. Separate the client's buttocks. Ask the client to take a deep breath. Gently insert the rectal tube 3 to 4 inches toward the umbilicus (2–3 inches for a child).	☐	☐	☐	_____

RECOMMENDED TECHNIQUE (*Continued*)	E	S	NP	Comments
12. Hold the tube in place with one hand while opening the clamp with the other hand. Allow solution to flow slowly into the rectum, while holding the can approximately 18 inches above the rectum. Enema should be delivered for 5 to 10 minutes. If the client complains of cramping, lower the bag or temporarily clamp the tubing.	☐	☐	☐	_____
13. Apply the clamp and remove the rectal tube when the enema is completed or when the client is unable to take more solution. Ask the client to retain the solution for as long as possible.	☐	☐	☐	_____
14. Assist the client into the bathroom or onto the bedpan with the head of the bed elevated. Place the call bell within easy reach.	☐	☐	☐	_____
15. When the client has expelled the enema solution, assist him or her back to bed or off the bedpan. Inspect the enema's results and obtain a specimen, if ordered.	☐	☐	☐	_____
16. Return the client to a comfortable position. Lower the bed, and raise the side rail.	☐	☐	☐	_____
17. Remove gloves and wash hands.	☐	☐	☐	_____
18. Document enema results and type of enema administered on the flow sheet or chart.	☐	☐	☐	_____

KEY: E = Excels   S = Satisfactory   NP = Needs Practice

☐ **Pass**   ☐ **Fail**

Student's Signature: _____ Date: _____

Instructor's Signature: _____ Date: _____

Measuring Urinary Output

SUPPLIES AND EQUIPMENT
✔ Gloves
✔ Graduated measuring container
✔ Bedpan, urinal, or toilet hat (half pan)

RECOMMENDED TECHNIQUE	E	S	NP	Comments
1. Wash hands and put on clean gloves.	☐	☐	☐	_____
2. Ask the client to void in the bedpan, toilet hat, or urinal. Label the hat, urinal, or bedpan with the client's name if he or she is sharing a room or several clients share the same toilet. Position the toilet hat in the toilet with the collecting receptacle toward the front.	☐	☐	☐	_____
3. Pour the urine into the graduated measuring container, and read the urine volume in milliliters.	☐	☐	☐	_____
4. Pour the urine into the toilet and flush, unless the urine is to be saved.	☐	☐	☐	_____
5. Rinse the bedpan or urinal and the measuring graduate in cool water.	☐	☐	☐	_____
6. Encourage the client to wash his or her hands.	☐	☐	☐	_____
7. Remove and dispose gloves and wash hands.	☐	☐	☐	_____
8. Record the urine volume on the output sheet.	☐	☐	☐	_____

KEY: E = Excels   S = Satisfactory   NP = Needs Practice

☐ **Pass**   ☐ **Fail**

Student's Signature: _____ Date: _____

Instructor's Signature: _____ Date: _____

Collecting a Urine Specimen From a Retention Catheter (Syringe and Needle System)

SUPPLIES AND EQUIPMENT

✔ Gloves
✔ Laboratory request slip
✔ Clamp or rubber band
✔ Container with label

✔ 10- to 20-mL syringe with 21- to 25-gauge needle
✔ Biohazard bag for transportation of specimen
✔ Alcohol prep or disinfectant swab

RECOMMENDED TECHNIQUE	E	S	NP	Comments
1. Gather supplies. Label the container.	☐	☐	☐	_____
2. Explain the procedure to the client.	☐	☐	☐	_____
3. Wash hands and put on gloves.	☐	☐	☐	_____
4. Clamp the drainage tubing or bend the tubing and secure it with a rubber band below the collection port. Allow adequate time for urine collection but no longer than 15 minutes.	☐	☐	☐	_____
5. Cleanse the aspiration port with an antiseptic swab, such as an alcohol prep.	☐	☐	☐	_____
6. Insert the needle into the aspiration port, and withdraw urine into the syringe. The laboratory test determines the amount of urine to collect.	☐	☐	☐	_____
7. Transfer the urine to the labeled specimen container. The container must be sterile for a culture and clean for a routine urinalysis.	☐	☐	☐	_____
8. Unclamp the catheter.	☐	☐	☐	_____
9. Prepare the container according to the agency's policy for transport to the laboratory.	☐	☐	☐	_____
10. Dispose of used equipment. Remove gloves and wash your hands.	☐	☐	☐	_____
11. Send the container to the laboratory immediately.	☐	☐	☐	_____
12. Document on the flow sheet, or record that you obtained the specimen.	☐	☐	☐	_____

KEY: E = Excels   S = Satisfactory   NP = Needs Practice

☐ **Pass**   ☐ **Fail**

Student's Signature: _____ Date: _____

Instructor's Signature: _____ Date: _____

Applying Antiembolism Stockings (TED Socks)

SUPPLIES AND EQUIPMENT
✔ Support stockings
✔ Talcum powder
✔ Tape measure

RECOMMENDED TECHNIQUE	E	S	NP	Comments
1. Explain the procedure to the client.	☐	☐	☐	_____
2. Use the tape measure to determine proper stocking size for the client.	☐	☐	☐	_____
3. Gather supplies.	☐	☐	☐	_____
4. Wash hands. Wear gloves if skin or the client's skin is not intact.	☐	☐	☐	_____
5. Assist the client to the supine position. Allow at least 15 minutes before applying stockings if the client has had the lower extremities in a dependent position.	☐	☐	☐	_____
6. Apply a small amount of talcum powder to the client's feet and legs if not contraindicated.	☐	☐	☐	_____
7. Grasp the stocking's heel, and turn it inside out.	☐	☐	☐	_____
8. Slip the client's foot, toes, and heel into the stocking. Center the heel in the stocking's heel pocket. Slide the stocking over the client's foot.	☐	☐	☐	_____
9. Support the client's ankle, and ease the stocking smoothly over the calf and remainder of the leg.	☐	☐	☐	_____
10. Pull forward slightly on the stocking's toe section.	☐	☐	☐	
11. Instruct the client to report any extreme discomfort.	☐	☐	☐	
12. Remove gloves (if worn) and wash hands.	☐	☐	☐	
13. Document the procedure on the client's record.	☐	☐	☐	

KEY: E = Excels   S = Satisfactory   NP = Needs Practice

☐ **Pass**   ☐ **Fail**

Student's Signature: _____ Date: _____

Instructor's Signature: _____ Date: _____

Using a Pulse Oximeter

SUPPLIES AND EQUIPMENT
✔ Pulse oximeter machine
✔ Sensor finger clip
✔ Nail polish remover (if needed)

RECOMMENDED TECHNIQUE	E	S	NP	Comments
1. Choose the sensor appropriate for the client's size.	☐	☐	☐	_____
2. Choose the appropriate location. Place the adhesive sensors and finger clip sensor for adults on their index, middle, or ring finger. Adhesive sensors may be placed on a client's toe unless the client has decreased circulation in the lower extremities. A small earlobe clip is available for use on small adults, children, and infants. Place the newborn adhesive sensor on the baby's foot.	☐	☐	☐	_____
3. Before applying the sensor, use an alcohol wipe on the site.	☐	☐	☐	_____
4. Remove any fingernail polish or acrylic nails on the fingers to be used.	☐	☐	☐	_____
5. If there are any doubts about the chosen site, check the client's proximal pulse and capillary refill. Check capillary refill by pressing on the client's skin. Normal color should return immediately when you release pressure.	☐	☐	☐	_____
6. Check the sensor's markings to make sure the light-emitting diode and photo detector are correctly aligned. They should be opposite each other.	☐	☐	☐	_____
7. Attach the sensor to the client cable and turn it on. There should be a digital read out or light bar to show readings and alarm settings. The type will depend on the facility's monitor.	☐	☐	☐	_____
8. Always make sure the alarms are on before leaving the client. The monitors come with preset limits that can be changed per physician's order or facility's policy. If the monitor is turned off, the alarm limits will default back to the original settings. The pulse oximeter gives audible and visual alarms. The audible alarm can be silenced for 60 seconds at a time by pressing "audio alarm off." It will reset after 60 seconds.	☐	☐	☐	_____

RECOMMENDED TECHNIQUE (*Continued*)	E	S	NP	Comments
9. Move an adhesive sensor every 4 hours and clip type every 2 hours.	☐	☐	☐	_____
10. Watch for signs of tissue breakdown or irritation from adhesives or clips.	☐	☐	☐	_____
11. Document the oximeter readings and location of sensor.	☐	☐	☐	_____
12. Notify instructor or team leader of any changes in readings of more than 5%.	☐	☐	☐	_____

KEY: E = Excels   S = Satisfactory   NP = Needs Practice

☐ **Pass**   ☐ **Fail**

Student's Signature: _____ Date: _____

Instructor's Signature: _____ Date: _____

Opening a Sterile Package

SUPPLIES AND EQUIPMENT
✔ Sterile supplies (as needed for procedure)
✔ Waist-high table

RECOMMENDED TECHNIQUE	E	S	NP	Comments
1. Gather supplies. Check the expiration date on sterile supplies.	☐	☐	☐	_____
2. Wash hands.	☐	☐	☐	_____
3. Explain the procedure to the client.	☐	☐	☐	_____
4. Prepare a waist-high working area.	☐	☐	☐	_____
5. Place the sterile package on the working area. Remove the outer covering or plastic wrap if present.	☐	☐	☐	_____
6. Grasp the edge of the outermost flap, and open the package away from you toward the back of the table.	☐	☐	☐	_____
7. Fold each side flap down toward the table. While holding the underside of the wrapper, push to bend it up in the middle, pulling the flaps tautly so that the flaps will not refold. Lay the package flat on the table.	☐	☐	☐	_____
8. Grasp the tip of the near flap and open it toward you. Pull the flap downward from underneath and pull it tautly into place.	☐	☐	☐	_____
9. Open any additional sterile packages without touching the contents.	☐	☐	☐	_____
10. Drop these items onto the sterile field.	☐	☐	☐	_____

KEY: E = Excels   S = Satisfactory   NP = Needs Practice

☐ **Pass**   ☐ **Fail**

Student's Signature: _____ Date: _____

Instructor's Signature: _____ Date: _____

Putting on Sterile Gloves

SUPPLIES AND EQUIPMENT
✔ Sterile gloves of the appropriate size

RECOMMENDED TECHNIQUE	E	S	NP	Comments
1. Wash hands.	☐	☐	☐	_____
2. Following Nursing Procedure 57-1, open the outer glove package on a clean, dry, flat surface at waist level or higher.	☐	☐	☐	_____
3. If there is an inner package, open it in the same way, keeping the sterile gloves on the inside surface with cuffs toward you.	☐	☐	☐	_____
4. Use one hand to grasp the inside upper surface of the glove's cuff for the opposite hand. Lift the glove up, and clear it of the wrapper.	☐	☐	☐	_____
5. Insert the opposite hand into the glove, placing the thumb and fingers in the proper openings. Pull the glove into place, touching only the inside of the cuff. Leave the cuff in place.	☐	☐	☐	_____
6. Slip the fingers of the sterile gloved hand under (inside) the cuff of the remaining glove while keeping the thumb pointed outward.	☐	☐	☐	_____
7. Lift the glove up, and clear it of the wrapper.	☐	☐	☐	_____
8. a. Insert the ungloved hand into the glove.	☐	☐	☐	_____
b. Pull the second glove on, touching *only* the outside of the sterile glove with the other sterile gloved hand and keeping the fingers inside the cuff.	☐	☐	☐	_____
c. Adjust gloves and snap cuffs into place. Avoid touching the inside glove and wrist areas.	☐	☐	☐	_____
9. Keep the sterile gloved hands above waist level. Make sure not to touch the clothes. Keep hands folded when not performing a procedure.	☐	☐	☐	_____

KEY: E = Excels   S = Satisfactory   NP = Needs Practice

☐ **Pass**   ☐ **Fail**

Student's Signature: _____ Date: _____

Instructor's Signature: _____ Date: _____

Catheterizing the Female Client

SUPPLIES AND EQUIPMENT

✔ Sterile catheterization tray containing sterile supplies:
    Gloves
    Basin
    Cotton balls
    Antiseptic solution and cup
    Straight or indwelling catheter (size appropriate for client)
    Lubricant (unless the catheter is prelubricated)
    Forceps
    Drapes (plain and fenestrated, containing an opening or window)
    Syringe prefilled with water or saline
    Specimen container

✔ Urine collection bag (may be attached to catheter)
✔ Flashlight or additional lamp
✔ Plastic biohazard bag
✔ Waterproof pad
✔ Velcro™ leg strap or nonallergenic tape (optional)
✔ Bath blanket
✔ Clean gloves, soap, and water
✔ Washcloth and towel

RECOMMENDED TECHNIQUE	E	S	NP	Comments
1. Explain the procedure to the client.	☐	☐	☐	_____
2. Gather supplies after checking the physician's order for catheterization.	☐	☐	☐	_____
3. Wash hands.	☐	☐	☐	_____
4. Close the door or pull the bed curtain. Adjust the bed to a comfortable working height. If right-handed, stand on the client's right side (if left handed, stand on the client's left side).	☐	☐	☐	_____
5. Assist the woman into a supine position with her feet spread apart and flat on the mattress and her knees flexed. Use a bath blanket to drape the client.	☐	☐	☐	_____
6. Put on clean gloves.	☐	☐	☐	_____
7. Wash the woman's perineal area with soap and water. Rinse and dry the area.	☐	☐	☐	_____
8. Remove the clean gloves, and wash hands again.	☐	☐	☐	_____
9. Ensure adequate lighting. Position a lamp at the foot of the bed, or another nurse may hold a flashlight.	☐	☐	☐	_____
10. Raise the bedside table to waist height. Open the sterile catheterization tray on the bedside table using appropriate sterile technique.	☐	☐	☐	_____
11. Put on sterile gloves.	☐	☐	☐	_____

RECOMMENDED TECHNIQUE (*Continued*)	E	S	NP	Comments

12. Pick up the sterile drape and gently shake it open. Grasp the upper corners and fold the drape back over the sterile gloves, making a cuff. ☐ ☐ ☐ _____

13. Keep the hands inside the cuff. ☐ ☐ ☐ _____

14. Ask the client to lift her buttocks. Place the drape between her thighs with the upper edge under her buttocks. ☐ ☐ ☐ _____

15. Set up equipment on the open sterile tray:

   a. Place the cotton balls into the cup. Open the package containing antiseptic, and pour it over the cotton balls. ☐ ☐ ☐ _____

   b. Remove the plastic covering from the catheter. For an indwelling catheter, attach the prefilled syringe to the balloon inflation port, and inflate the balloon with the appropriate amount of fluid to test the balloon. After the balloon inflates, aspirate the fluid back into the syringe, leaving the syringe connected to the port and the balloon deflated. ☐ ☐ ☐ _____

   c. Open the lubricant, and lubricate the catheter's tip 1 to 2 inches. Leave the catheter tip inside the sterile lubricant package until needed. ☐ ☐ ☐ _____

   d. Unscrew the cap from the specimen container if a specimen is ordered. ☐ ☐ ☐ _____

   e. If a straight catheter is being used, position the drainage end of the catheter in the basin to catch the urine. ☐ ☐ ☐ _____

16. Move the catheterization tray with the equipment onto the sterile drape between the client's thighs. ☐ ☐ ☐ _____

17. While using the nondominant hand, separate and gently spread the woman's labia minora to expose her urinary meatus. Keep this hand in this position. ☐ ☐ ☐ _____

18. With the dominant hand, use the forceps to pick up cotton balls. Cleanse both labial folds and then the meatus. Use a new cotton ball for each stroke, moving from top to bottom (front to back). Discard each used cotton ball in the plastic biohazard bag. Cleanse the meatus last. (Rationale: Moving from clean to dirty lessens the chance of introducing microorganisms into the client's bladder. Using a new cotton ball each time helps to keep the area as clean as possible.) ☐ ☐ ☐ _____

RECOMMENDED TECHNIQUE (*Continued*)	E	S	NP	Comments
19. Pick up the catheter approximately 3 inches from the tip with the dominant hand. Place the drainage end in the basin to catch the urine flow (or if a specimen is to be obtained, place the drainage end into the specimen container). If the catheter is indwelling, it may already be attached to the drainage tubing.	☐	☐	☐	_____
20. Ask the client to breathe deeply and slowly through her mouth. Insert the catheter gently into the urinary meatus advancing it 2 to 3 inches until urine begins to drain. If the catheter is in dwelling, advance it another 1 to 2 inches. Never force insertion of the catheter if resistance is felt. Move the non-dominant hand to hold the catheter in place between two fingers, bracing the rest of this hand against the client's perineum. Collect a urine specimen if one is ordered.	☐	☐	☐	_____
21. If the catheter is not to be indwelling, allow urine to drain into the basin. Remove the catheter after urine has drained. For an indwelling catheter, inject the fluid to inflate the balloon. Pull gently on the catheter to check that the balloon is inflated and that the catheter is secure.	☐	☐	☐	_____
22. Use a leg strap or tape to anchor the tubing from the indwelling catheter. Position the drainage bag below bladder level. The catheter should pass over the woman's leg.	☐	☐	☐	_____
23. Dry the client's perineal area if necessary. Measure the urine amount.	☐	☐	☐	_____
24. Remove gloves. Reposition and cover the client. Lower the bed. Remove equipment.	☐	☐	☐	_____
25. Dispose of equipment according to agency policy.	☐	☐	☐	_____
26. Dispose of gloves.	☐	☐	☐	_____
27. Wash hands.	☐	☐	☐	_____
28. Document the size and type of catheter inserted and the client's response. Record the amount of urine obtained, its appearance, and specimen collection if one was obtained.	☐	☐	☐	_____

KEY: E = Excels   S = Satisfactory   NP = Needs Practice

☐ **Pass**   ☐ **Fail**

Student's Signature: _____ Date: _____

Instructor's Signature: _____ Date: _____

Catheterizing the Male Client

SUPPLIES AND EQUIPMENT
Same as for "Catheterizing the Female Patient" (see Nursing Procedure 57-3).

RECOMMENDED TECHNIQUE	E	S	NP	Comments
1. Follow steps 1 through 4 in Nursing Procedure 57-3.	☐	☐	☐	_____
2. Assist the man to lie on his back with his legs slightly apart. Position the drape or bath blanket so only the penis is uncovered.	☐	☐	☐	_____
3. Put on clean gloves.	☐	☐	☐	_____
4. Wash the penis with soap and water. Rinse and dry.	☐	☐	☐	_____
5. Remove the gloves and wash the hands again.	☐	☐	☐	_____
6. Open the sterile catheterization tray on the bedside table.	☐	☐	☐	_____
7. Put on sterile gloves. Pick up the sterile drape, shake it open, and lay it on the client's thighs. Place the opening of the fenestrated drape over the man's penis.	☐	☐	☐	_____
8. Set up the equipment on the tray, the same as for a female client (see Nursing Procedure 57-3).	☐	☐	☐	_____
9. Lubricate the catheter tip for male catheterization 5 to 7 inches (sometimes lubricant is instilled directly into the urethra).	☐	☐	☐	_____
10. Move the catheterization tray onto the sterile drape.	☐	☐	☐	_____
11. Use nondominant hand to grasp the penis. If the client is uncircumcised, retract his foreskin before cleansing. With the forceps, pick up a cotton ball, and cleanse from the meatus outward in a circular motion. Repeat three times, using each cotton ball only once.	☐	☐	☐	_____
12. Pick up the catheter approximately 3 inches from the tip with your dominant hand. Place the drainage end in the basin. If the catheter is indwelling, it may already be attached to drainage tubing.	☐	☐	☐	_____
13. Lift the penis to an upright perpendicular position. Gently pressing the end of the penis from two sides may help to open the meatus. Ask the client to bear down as if voiding.	☐	☐	☐	_____

RECOMMENDED TECHNIQUE (*Continued*)	E	S	NP	Comments
14. Insert the catheter gently into the meatus, advancing it 7 to 9 inches or until urine begins to drain. If resistance is encountered when passing the catheter, rotate it slightly or withdraw it, rather than forcing it.	☐	☐	☐	_____
15. For an indwelling catheter, advance it another inch. Collect a urine specimen if one is ordered.	☐	☐	☐	_____
16. Make the following exceptions for the male client:	☐	☐	☐	_____
a. Tape or secure the catheter to his lower abdomen or upper thigh, allowing some slack in the tubing.	☐	☐	☐	_____
b. Return the foreskin to its original position in the uncircumcised man.	☐	☐	☐	_____
17. Position the drainage bag below bladder level.	☐	☐	☐	_____
18. Dry the client's perineal area if necessary. Measure the urine amount.	☐	☐	☐	_____
19. Remove gloves. Reposition and cover the client. Lower the bed. Remove equipment.	☐	☐	☐	_____
20. Dispose of equipment according to agency policy.	☐	☐	☐	_____
21. Dispose of gloves.	☐	☐	☐	_____
22. Wash the hands.	☐	☐	☐	_____
23. Document the size and type of catheter inserted and the client's response. Record the amount of urine obtained, its appearance, and specimen collection if one was obtained.	☐	☐	☐	_____

KEY: E = Excels   S = Satisfactory   NP = Needs Practice

☐ **Pass**   ☐ **Fail**

Student's Signature: _____   Date: _____

Instructor's Signature: _____   Date: _____

Removing the Retention Catheter

SUPPLIES AND EQUIPMENT
✔ Gloves
✔ Waterproof pad
✔ Syringe (size is determined by volume of fluid used to inflate balloon)
✔ Soap, water, washcloth, and towel

RECOMMENDED TECHNIQUE	E	S	NP	Comments
1. Explain the procedure to the client.	☐	☐	☐	_____
2. Gather supplies after checking the physician's order for catheter removal.	☐	☐	☐	_____
3. Wash hands and put on gloves.	☐	☐	☐	_____
4. Close the door or pull the bed curtains. Adjust the bed to a comfortable working height. Place a waterproof pad between the client's thighs.	☐	☐	☐	_____
5. Attach the syringe's hub to inflation port, or insert a needleless hub. Deflate the balloon by completely aspirating all the fluid. *Never* cut a catheter.	☐	☐	☐	_____
6. Pull the catheter out gently and slowly.	☐	☐	☐	_____
7. Wrap the catheter in a waterproof pad. Remove the catheter, drainage bag, and equipment from the bedside, disposing according to agency policy.	☐	☐	☐	_____
8. Measure urine in the drainage bag, and record findings on the intake and output form.	☐	☐	☐	_____
9. Assist the client to cleanse and dry the perineal area. Return the client to a position of comfort.	☐	☐	☐	_____
10. Remove gloves and wash hands.	☐	☐	☐	_____
11. Document catheter removal on the appropriate form.	☐	☐	☐	_____

KEY: E = Excels S = Satisfactory NP = Needs Practice

☐ **Pass**   ☐ **Fail**

Student's Signature: _____ Date: _____

Instructor's Signature: _____ Date: _____

Changing a Dry Sterile Dressing

SUPPLIES AND EQUIPMENT
- ✔ Clean gloves
- ✔ Plastic biohazard bag
- ✔ Abdominal (ABD) pads
- ✔ Sterile dressings, as ordered
- ✔ Sterile saline or water
- ✔ Bath blanket
- ✔ Sterile gloves
- ✔ Tape or Montgomery straps
- ✔ Waterproof pads
- ✔ Forceps from sterile suture removal set (optional)

RECOMMENDED TECHNIQUE	E	S	NP	Comments
1. Explain the procedure to the client.	☐	☐	☐	_____
2. Gather supplies after checking the physician's order for the dressing change.	☐	☐	☐	_____
3. Wash hands.	☐	☐	☐	_____
4. Close the door or pull the bed curtains. Assist the client to a comfortable position. Expose only the area to redress, using a bath blanket if necessary. Place a waterproof pad under the client to protect the bed.	☐	☐	☐	_____
5. Prepare a plastic biohazard bag as a receptacle for soiled dressings. Fold back the cuff, and place it within reach of your working area.	☐	☐	☐	_____
6. Put on clean gloves.	☐	☐	☐	_____
7. Untie the Montgomery straps, or gently loosen the tape.	☐	☐	☐	_____
8. Remove the soiled dressing, being careful not to tear the wound or dislodge any drains. Use sterile saline to moisten the dressing if it is sticking to the wound.	☐	☐	☐	_____
9. Lift the soiled side of the dressing away from the client's view.	☐	☐	☐	_____
10. Assess the amount, color, odor, and consistency of the drainage. Observe the wound and surrounding tissues. Measure the wound.	☐	☐	☐	_____
11. Remove gloves and place them in the plastic bag.	☐	☐	☐	_____
12. Wash hands.	☐	☐	☐	_____
13. Prepare a sterile field on the bedside table, and open sterile dressings onto it.	☐	☐	☐	_____
14. Uncap the sterile saline or other ordered solution to cleanse the wound. Place additional sterile dressings or swabs for cleansing onto the sterile field.	☐	☐	☐	_____

RECOMMENDED TECHNIQUE (*Continued*)	E	S	NP	Comments
15. Put on sterile gloves.	☐	☐	☐	_____
16. Moisten sterile dressings or swabs and cleanse the wound, if ordered, moving from top to bottom or from the center of the wound outward (may use forceps). Use a new swab or gauze pad for each cleansing motion. Do not use alcohol or soap.	☐	☐	☐	_____
17. If necessary, use a gauze pad to dry the wound.	☐	☐	☐	_____
18. Carefully inspect the wound. Be prepared to describe the wound accurately.	☐	☐	☐	_____
19. Apply any ointments or medications to the wound as ordered.	☐	☐	☐	_____
20. Apply a layer of dry sterile dressings over the incision and wound area. Pad with additional dressings, and cover with a sterile ABD pad, if required.	☐	☐	☐	_____
21. Remove gloves and place them in the disposal biohazard bag.	☐	☐	☐	_____
22. Wash hands.	☐	☐	☐	_____
23. Apply tape or tie dressing with Montgomery straps.	☐	☐	☐	_____
24. Reposition and cover the client while preventing pressure on the wound.	☐	☐	☐	_____
25. Handle only the outside of the biohazard bag, keeping hands inside the cuff and carefully closing it. Dispose of the bag with used supplies according to agency policy.	☐	☐	☐	_____
26. Wash hands.	☐	☐	☐	_____
27. Document wound care and all assessments of the wound and drainage.	☐	☐	☐	_____

KEY: E = Excels   S = Satisfactory   NP = Needs Practice

☐ **Pass**   ☐ **Fail**

Student's Signature: _____ Date: _____

Instructor's Signature: _____ Date: _____

Testing for Blood Glucose Level

SUPPLIES AND EQUIPMENT
- ✔ Blood glucose testing strips
- ✔ Glucose testing meter
- ✔ Sterile lancet
- ✔ Lancet activating device (optional)
- ✔ Cotton balls
- ✔ Alcohol swab
- ✔ Gloves

RECOMMENDED TECHNIQUE	E	S	NP	Comments
1. Wash hands.	☐	☐	☐	_____
2. Gather supplies.	☐	☐	☐	_____
3. Explain the procedure to the client.	☐	☐	☐	_____
4. Have the client wash his or her hands with warm water.	☐	☐	☐	_____
5. Assist the client to a comfortable position.	☐	☐	☐	_____
6. Remove a test strip from the container. Turn on the glucose testing meter. Check that the code number on the strip matches the code number that appears initially on the monitor screen (or follow the manufacturer's instructions).	☐	☐	☐	_____
7. Prepare the lancet by twisting off the cap. Arm the automatic device by pushing back the plunger until it clicks. Attach the lancet. Remove the cap. Keep the tip sterile.	☐	☐	☐	_____
8. Put on gloves.	☐	☐	☐	_____
9. Select the site on the client's finger for puncture. Gently massage the finger toward the intended puncture site, keeping the finger in dependent position.	☐	☐	☐	_____
10. Clean the site with alcohol prep, and allow the area to dry thoroughly. (Clients may omit this step at home.)	☐	☐	☐	_____
11. Prick the side of the client's finger with a lancet and squeeze gently. Use a cotton ball to wipe away the first drop of blood if recommended for the particular meter.	☐	☐	☐	_____
12. Gently touch the drop of blood to the strip's target area, or use a pipette as instructed. Have the client hold a clean cotton ball to the puncture site for a few seconds.	☐	☐	☐	_____
13. Insert the strip as far as it will go into the meter with the target area facing the red dot on the meter (or follow manufacturer's directions for specific meter).	☐	☐	☐	_____

RECOMMENDED TECHNIQUE (*Continued*)	E	S	NP	Comments
14. Read test results in 15 to 60 seconds on the meter face. Remove the strip and turn off the meter.	☐	☐	☐	_____
15. Dispose of equipment properly. Remove gloves and wash hands.	☐	☐	☐	_____
16. Record blood glucose reading on proper forms. Check to see if the client is on insulin coverage.	☐	☐	☐	_____

KEY: E = Excels   S = Satisfactory   NP = Needs Practice

☐ **Pass**   ☐ **Fail**

Student's Signature: _____   Date: _____

Instructor's Signature: _____   Date: _____

Supplying Oxygen With the Nasal Cannula

SUPPLIES AND EQUIPMENT

✔ Flow meter
✔ Oxygen source
✔ Nasal cannula and tubing

✔ Humidifier and sterile water (optional)
✔ Oxygen-in-use sign ("No Smoking")
✔ Gloves

RECOMMENDED TECHNIQUE	E	S	NP	Comments
1. Check the physician's orders.	☐	☐	☐	_____
2. Gather supplies.	☐	☐	☐	_____
3. Wash hands. Put on gloves.	☐	☐	☐	_____
4. Explain the procedure to the client.	☐	☐	☐	_____
5. Prepare the oxygen equipment:				
a. Plug the flow meter into the wall outlet or oxygen tank.	☐	☐	☐	_____
b. Attach the humidifier to the flow meter.	☐	☐	☐	_____
c. Fill the humidifier with sterile water.	☐	☐	☐	_____
d. Attach the cannula with the connecting tubing to the adapter on the humidifier.	☐	☐	☐	_____
6. Adjust the flow meter's setting to the ordered flow rate. Check that oxygen is flowing out of the prongs. The flow rate through the cannula should not exceed 6 LPM.	☐	☐	☐	_____
7. Insert the prongs into the client's nostrils. Adjust the tubing behind the client's ears and slide the plastic adapter under the client's chin until he or she is comfortable.	☐	☐	☐	_____
8. Encourage the client to breathe through the nose rather than the mouth.	☐	☐	☐	_____
9. Assess the client's comfort level. Leave the call signal within reach.	☐	☐	☐	_____
10. Dispose of gloves and wash hands.	☐	☐	☐	_____
11. Place "No Smoking" sign at entry into the room.	☐	☐	☐	_____
12. Document the procedure, and record the client's reaction.	☐	☐	☐	_____
13. Check the oxygen setup, including the water level in the humidifier. Clean the cannula, and assess the client's nares at least every 8 hours.	☐	☐	☐	_____

Suctioning and Providing Tracheostomy Care

SUPPLIES AND EQUIPMENT

✔ Tracheostomy suctioning kit containing the following sterile supplies:
  Gloves
  Suction catheter
  Basins or containers
  Sterile normal saline
  Portable or wall suction apparatus

Sterile tracheostomy dressing
Twill tape or Velcro™ trach ties
Hydrogen peroxide
Sterile gauze pads
Disposable inner cannula (optional)
✔ Goggles and gown (optional)
✔ Clean towel or plastic drape (optional)

RECOMMENDED TECHNIQUE	E	S	NP	Comments
1. Check the physician's order.	☐	☐	☐	_____
2. Gather supplies.	☐	☐	☐	_____
3. Explain the procedure to the client.	☐	☐	☐	_____
4. Wash hands.	☐	☐	☐	_____
5. Adjust bed to a comfortable working height.	☐	☐	☐	_____
6. Assist the conscious client to a semi- or high-Fowler's position. Place the unconscious client on his or her side, facing the nurse.	☐	☐	☐	_____
7. Place a towel or drape across the client's chest. Put on a gown or goggles (optional). Turn on suction to the appropriate level. Put on gloves.	☐	☐	☐	_____
8. Prepare the suction equipment:	☐	☐	☐	_____
a. Open the sterile tracheostomy suctioning kit and cleaning supplies on the bedside tray or table.	☐	☐	☐	_____
b. Pick up the sterile container, open it, and pour sterile saline into it.	☐	☐	☐	_____
c. Put on sterile gloves.	☐	☐	☐	_____
d. Pick up the sterile suction catheter with dominant hand.	☐	☐	☐	_____
e. Use nondominant hand to connect the wall or portable suction catheter tubing to the sterile suction catheter.	☐	☐	☐	_____

KEY: E = Excels S = Satisfactory NP = Needs Practice

☐ **Pass** ☐ **Fail**

Student's Signature: _____ Date: _____
Instructor's Signature: _____ Date: _____

RECOMMENDED TECHNIQUE (*Continued*)	E	S	NP	Comments
9. Dip the suction catheter into the basin with sterile saline. Use the thumb on non-dominant hand to occlude the suction port.	☐	☐	☐	_____
10. Remove the oxygen delivery system with the nondominant hand.	☐	☐	☐	_____
11. Use the dominant hand to insert the catheter into the trachea for 4 to 5 inches or until the client coughs. Do not apply suction while inserting the catheter.	☐	☐	☐	_____
12. Occlude the suction port with the non-dominant thumb while rotating and removing the catheter. Suctioning should not continue for longer than 10-second intervals.	☐	☐	☐	_____
13. Dip the catheter into saline solution while applying the suction. Repeat the suctioning procedure if necessary. Allow 1 minute between suctioning. Reapply the oxygen delivery system while waiting to continue the procedure.	☐	☐	☐	_____
14. Before removing gloves, cleanse the cannula. If the inner cannula is disposable, remove and replace it with a clean cannula. For the replaceable cannula:	☐	☐	☐	_____
a. Unlock the cannula and carefully remove it.	☐	☐	☐	_____
b. Hold it over the sterile basin.	☐	☐	☐	_____
c. Rinse it with sterile saline.	☐	☐	☐	_____
d. Gently replace the inner cannula and lock it in place.	☐	☐	☐	_____
15. Cleanse around the tracheostomy stoma and under the tracheostomy tube faceplate with sterile cotton-tipped swabs dipped in hydrogen peroxide.	☐	☐	☐	_____
16. Rinse the area using cotton-tipped swabs moistened in normal saline.	☐	☐	☐	_____
17. Dry the area with a dry sterile gauze pad.	☐	☐	☐	_____
18. Change the tracheostomy tube tape if necessary:	☐	☐	☐	_____
a. Have an assistant hold the tracheostomy tube in place with a sterile hand. If unassisted, leave the soiled tapes in place until new ones are inserted and secured.	☐	☐	☐	_____

RECOMMENDED TECHNIQUE (*Continued*)   **E   S   NP   Comments**

b. Pass the ends of the tape through the opening on the faceplate, and bring them behind the client's neck to the other opening on the opposite side of the faceplate.   ☐   ☐   ☐   _____

c. Insert tape through the opening; pull securely, and tie or Velcro™ into place.   ☐   ☐   ☐   _____

d. If necessary, remove the soiled tape.   ☐   ☐   ☐   _____

19. Place a sterile tracheostomy dressing under the faceplate. Tegaderm also may be applied under the gauze.   ☐   ☐   ☐   _____

20. Reattach the oxygen delivery system over the tracheostomy tube.   ☐   ☐   ☐   _____

21. Remove gloves by pulling the glove over the suction catheter; also remove goggles and gown (if worn). Reposition the client. Lower the bed.   ☐   ☐   ☐   _____

22. Wash hands.   ☐   ☐   ☐   _____

23. Dispose of equipment according to agency's policy.   ☐   ☐   ☐   _____

24. Document the suctioning procedure, nature and amount of secretions, and the client's response. Record respiratory assessments following suctioning procedure.   ☐   ☐   ☐   _____

25. Replace bed to its lowest level. Ensure that side rails are up and call light is with client's easy reach.   ☐   ☐   ☐   _____

KEY: E = Excels   S = Satisfactory   NP = Needs Practice

☐ **Pass**   ☐ **Fail**

Student's Signature: _____ Date: _____

Instructor's Signature: _____ Date: _____

Changing the Ostomy Appliance

SUPPLIES AND EQUIPMENT

- ✔ Pouch or pattern
- ✔ Pouch adhesive wafer
- ✔ Closure clip
- ✔ Stomahesive paste (optional)
- ✔ Cotton balls or gauze
- ✔ Scissors
- ✔ Pen or pencil
- ✔ Tissues
- ✔ Water
- ✔ Soft towel
- ✔ Liquid deodorant
- ✔ Plastic waste bag
- ✔ Gloves

RECOMMENDED TECHNIQUE	E	S	NP	Comments
1. Wash hands and apply gloves.	☐	☐	☐	_____
2. Arrange all needed equipment within the client's reach.	☐	☐	☐	_____
3. Teach the client to cuff (turn back) the tail of the pouch before emptying. Empty the old appliance into the toilet and flush.	☐	☐	☐	_____
4. Locate the stoma size pattern. With a pen, trace this size hole on the paper backing of the pouch adhesive. Cut out the opening.	☐	☐	☐	_____
5. Remove the paper backing from the pouch adhesive (wafer). Apply a thin bead of Stomahesive paste to the edge of the cut adhesive.	☐	☐	☐	_____
6. Remove the old appliance gently, and wipe around the stoma with tissue.	☐	☐	☐	_____
7. Dispose of the old appliance in a plastic bag. Save the closure clip.	☐	☐	☐	_____
8. Inspect the skin. Wash the area with warm water; do not use soap.	☐	☐	☐	_____
9. Dry the skin carefully. Apply the new appliance. Hold in place for 2 minutes.	☐	☐	☐	_____
10. Add a few drops of the deodorant to the pouch, and clamp it closed.	☐	☐	☐	_____
11. Dispose of waste material and gloves.	☐	☐	☐	_____
12. Wash hands.	☐	☐	☐	_____
13. Document the procedure, noting the client's reactions.	☐	☐	☐	_____

KEY: E = Excels   S = Satisfactory   NP = Needs Practice

☐ **Pass**   ☐ **Fail**

Student's Signature: _____ Date: _____

Instructor's Signature: _____ Date: _____